How to Grow Glorious Wheatgrass at Home Tutorial

With Salty Sea Mineral Eco-Fertilization for Superior Mineral Rich Soil

Eryn Paige

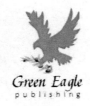

Green Eagle
publishing

Copyright Notice

How to Grow Glorious Wheatgrass at Home Tutorial

Published by

Green Eagle Publishing

ISBN-13: 978-0615766379

Visit the author at:

www.HealthBanquet.com

www.facebook.com/HealthBanquet

www.twitter.com/HealthBanquet

Sign up for Eryn's free Health Banquet Digest newsletter at www.HealthBanquet.com

Terms of Use & Disclaimer

Special Terms of Use:

Disclaimer: This How *To Grow Glorious Wheatgrass At Home Tutorial - With Salty Sea Mineral Eco-Fertilization for Superior Mineral Rich Soil* is not intended to be a prescription for the user. This digital tutorial does not offer medical advice and its content has not been evaluated by the US Food and Drug Administration. It simply presents educational information regarding how to grow wheatgrass, and information pertaining to its characteristics. No information or products described in this tutorial should be relied upon to diagnose, treat, cure, or prevent disease.

Because there is always some risk involved, the author is not responsible for any adverse effects or consequences resulting from the use of any of the suggestions, preparations, or procedures in this tutorial. Please do not use this tutorial if you are unwilling to assume the risk. Always feel free to consult a physician or other qualified health professional. It is always good to work as a team with your health care practitioners. It is a sign of strength and wisdom to seek a second or third opinion.

Contraindications: Those on medications that are unable to take vegetables, or vegetables with higher amounts of vitamin K like wheatgrass, should check with their healthcare provider. Pregnant and nursing mothers should check with their doctor to find out if they support consuming wheatgrass juice. Wheatgrass contains no wheat gluten.

Highly recommended wheatgrass growing supplies are presented at the end of this tutorial and are available through the HealthBanquet.com Amazon store. HealthBanquet.com will receive a small commission.

Table of Contents

About the Author

Eryn Paige, Editor of HealthBanquet.com, enjoys researching and educating on nature's bounty—exquisite nature that is available to keep us healthier and happier on planet Earth. Her past experiences have led to the creation of this *How to Grow Glorious Wheatgrass at Home Tutorial - With Salty Sea Mineral Eco-Fertilization for Superior Mineral Rich Soil*. She is a wheatgrass aficionado.

Having personally experienced a health set-back later in life, she set out to get better, and uncovered valuable nutritional and wellness information that she knew she had to share to help others, and thus HealthBanquet.com, LLC was created. She learned of the late Dr. Weston A. Price, author of *Nutrition and Physical Degeneration*. From this enduring classic book, she discovered the superb health and healthy teeth the depicted peoples had that consumed replenishing foods from mineral rich soils. These peoples from around the world had beautiful physiques, and were lacking the serious health issues affecting growing numbers, of even the youngest children, in our population. She looks forward to raw milk dispensers providing safe raw milk from grass fed cows to the people in the United States, as is being done around the world.

Because of her particular passion for the phenomenal wheatgrass, she has been writing about wheatgrass juice, and answering questions about successfully growing wheatgrass for years at HealthBanquet.com, LLC. She remains in awe of the remarkable blood building capabilities of wheatgrass—an astounding plant bursting with potent nutrition, enzymes, liquid chlorophyll, and restorative minerals and trace elements.

Enchanted by its inherent life force igniting abilities that have revitalized the minds and physical bodies of so many, she would like you to know that wheatgrass juice *nutritional therapy* is being used around the world to support health, assist the ailing to rejuvenate and help restore their wellness. In fact, she would like to share that even Jesus Christ reportedly advocated its health benefits.

Dedication and Gratitude

This *How to Grow Glorious Wheatgrass at Home Tutorial - With Salty Sea Mineral Eco-Fertilization for Superior Mineral Rich Soil* is dedicated to all those wanting to grow glorious, incredibly nutritious wheatgrass, in the most simple way. It is for those looking to *better maintain* or *improve* their health—naturally and safely. It is also for all those "trapped in ailing bodies" and those looking for a *brighter* and *healthier* tomorrow. I hope understanding the important messages this tutorial conveys and incorporating fresh wheatgrass juice and healthy foods into the diet, will help one to move forward on the road back to wellness, so life can be more fully embraced once again. God bless you on this journey. . . . May you Replenish, Revive and RELIVE!

It is also dedicated in memory of Ann Wigmore, author of *The Wheatgrass Book*. It was because of Wigmore's unwavering belief in the exceptionally nutritive nature of wheatgrass, that people took notice and realized how *powerfully* beneficial it could be to drink, and be used externally as well. Additionally, this tutorial is dedicated in memory of the profound nutritional researcher, Dr. Weston A. Price, author of *Nutrition and Physical Degeneration*. Dr. Price precisely communicated his research on the impact that soil fertility and nutrition had on mankind's physical structure, behavior, overall health, and reproductive ability. He also observed the *increased* nutrients in the by-products of cows such as their milk, when the cows grazed on the marvelous young grasses, *particularly* wheat grass and other cereal grasses, grown on mineral rich soil. Importantly, it is also dedicated in memory of Dr. Maynard Murray, author of *Sea Energy Agriculture*. The time is now for his vision of sustainable and earth friendly sea energy agriculture to fully transpire.

Tremendous gratitude to my husband Mark whose support allowed me the needed time necessary to bring this wheatgrass growing tutorial to fruition. What I thought would be a brief tutorial, kept expanding, as I learned more and knew this information must be communicated.

Additionally, I would like to thank the following *very special* people for believing in me and this project; my nutrition-minded mother Donna who provided plenty of green drinks and satiating full-fat raw milk growing up and kept sweets to a minimum in our cupboards (a quality appreciated years later), and my mother-in-law Lucille and father-in-law Norman. In memory of my father, lots of gratitude for sharing his love of nature with me. Much appreciation to family members and good friends—*all* whom are truly the "wind beneath my wings."

Also, a big heartfelt thank you to all the natural health crusaders and healthy food advocates sharing traditional dietary principles including non-adulterated foods and good fats. Sincere appreciation to those ethical "salt of the earth" farmers "feeding their soils well," and incorporating organic and sustainable agricultural methods—so they can better "feed the world" at a time when it is needed most. Finally, much gratitude to all the incredible moms and dads around the world doing their best to make better nutritional choices for their children, so they will have healthier futures.

Request: After you have successfully grown your nutritious wheatgrass, would you please consider leaving a short review at Amazon?

Preface - 1

Welcome to the exciting world of wheatgrass growing. Not only is growing wheatgrass a lot of fun, but it is great to know that through its regular consumption, you can truly increase your important nutrient uptake, naturally. I will teach you how to *simply* grow beautiful and healthy wheatgrass, indoors in soil—which can be grown every single day of the year.

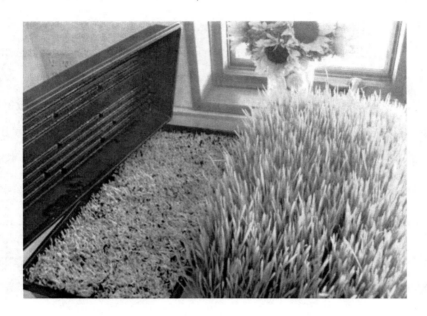

This tutorial lays out clear visual aids and step-by-step instructions on how to successfully grow glorious wheatgrass at home. It covers many wheatgrass growing topics including the importance of good wheat seed and nutritious soil, how to address mold, plus so much more. This information will help you bring forth even healthier wheatgrass, with improved germination.

This tutorial also answers the remaining questions I had after trying to learn how to successfully grow wheatgrass at home. **I recommend first reading through the entire tutorial, before starting to grow your wheatgrass, and before purchasing the supplies for growing your wheatgrass.**

> **"Celebrate this simple looking plant, that holds within it perhaps nature's greatest fountain of rejuvenation and powerful nourishment."**

I tried to keep this tutorial brief, and yet beneficially detailed, with the key information you need to optimally grow wheatgrass at home indoors. I have answered additional wheatgrass growing questions at my wheatgrass growing question and answer forum at HealthBanquet.com.

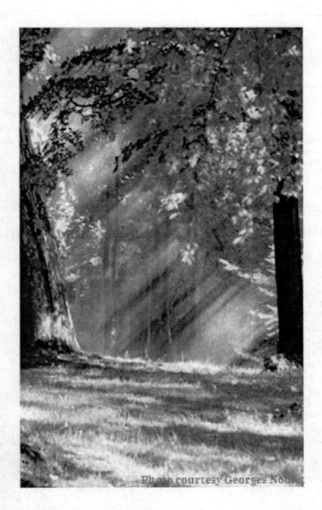

Photo courtesy Georges Noël

This growing wheatgrass tutorial complements the other wheatgrass books on the market. However, it specifically *zeros in* on the art of growing wheatgrass at home indoors and in soil. I wish this tutorial would have been available to me when I was first learning how to grow wheatgrass, as I would have found a more favorable outcome growing wheatgrass much sooner.

> **"Grass is the most valuable green food on our planet Earth."**

When it comes to powerful nutrition, I believe no single whole food source can beat fresh, organic, wheatgrass juice. After all, nutritious grass is what much of the animal kingdom thrives on. And I believe it is very important to pay close attention to Mother Nature and the wisdom she imparts.

> **"Wheatgrass is indeed humble like the grass beneath our feet, and yet mighty in its healing and replenishing abilities."**

Importantly, the *more* mineral rich the grass, the *healthier* the animal. And wheatgrass is the nourishing leader in the entire grass family. In terms of being supremely salubrious, it is unequivocally in a league of its own.

Because of my knowledge and personal experience growing and drinking wheatgrass juice, and based on questions I was receiving about wheatgrass growing, I knew I had to write this *How to Grow Glorious Wheatgrass at Home Tutorial*.

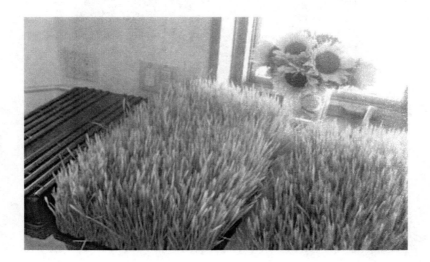

Even if you are already growing wheatgrass at home, I know you will pick up some additional very helpful tips and learn different methods to grow wheatgrass. I hope you enjoy experimenting with the *four* wheatgrass growing methods I share, to find *your* personal preference. Method One which I explain first in Chapter 6, is the most popular, and a great way to first start growing wheatgrass. I also really enjoy growing with Method Three explained in Chapter 9.

The wheatgrass growing steps and methods I present will lead you to great success growing your wheatgrass. Go ahead and later alter, if desired, your selected growing wheatgrass approach—taking your wheatgrass growing needs, preferences, and environment into consideration. You are in charge of your wheatgrass growing. Again, start out with Method One and you can branch out from there.

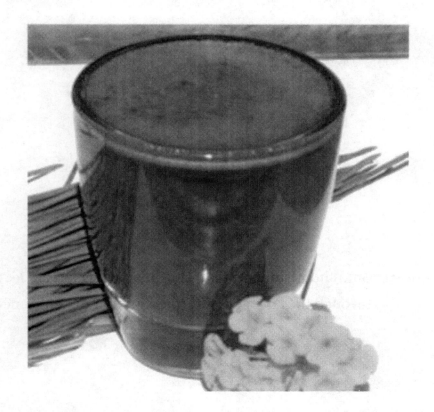

Now, let's have fun and learn how to grow wheatgrass so you can begin to experience its generous goodness, and its nutritious extract penetrate your very being....

Why I Grow and Drink Almighty Wheatgrass Juice

Wheatgrass growing is a wonderful part of my life. I slowly built up to consume about 1 - 2 ounces per day (some drink less per day), occasionally 3 ounces, and take a break now and then. Sometimes I drink it straight, sometimes I add water, and sometimes I mix it with a variety of other juiced fruits and vegetables. Some take more ounces per day based on their personal situation and preference. There are more detailed wheatgrass dosage recommendations at HealthBanquet.com.

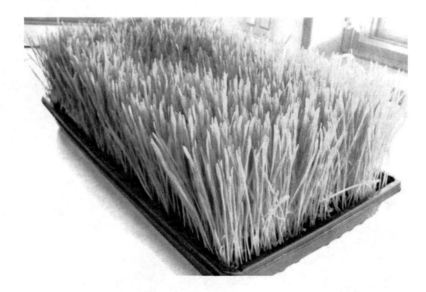

I enjoy the strength and nourishment that this marvelous green leafed vegetable provides. I seem to go through the day more effortlessly and more enlivened.

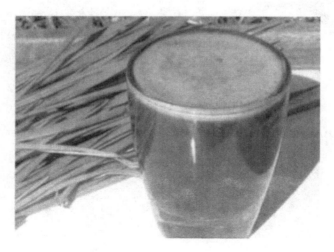

I consider it a way to help detoxify, remineralize, support bone and teeth health, support skin health, strengthen my immune system, help build healthier blood so it can more capably oxygenate and nourish me internally, support cellular health, plus so much more.

It benefits my entire body, as it circulates within. This nutrient packed plant feeds my body with its wide variety of valuable minerals and trace elements. I am happier and lighter feeling when I consume the wheatgrass juice. My body and mind takes on the positive energy of this restorative green beverage when I consume it. I feel everything within me operates better when I drink it.

I love seeing how the wheatgrass juice given to my friends and family transforms their lives in a good way. I discovered the power of wheatgrass juice on my personal journey to improve my health. Understanding its *tremendous* nourishing abilities and therapeutic potential, I incorporated it into my diet.

Why is Wheatgrass so Beneficial?

Since ancient times, because of the medicinal properties of wheatgrass, it has been traditionally used to help prevent and treat different disorders and diseases. This superb, raw, green, aqueous vegetable extract has been demonstrated to help protect DNA from free radicals, and contains potent *anti*-mutagenic characteristics. A mutagen is a physical or chemical agent that mutates or changes the genes of plants or animals. Many genetic mutations can cause cancer.

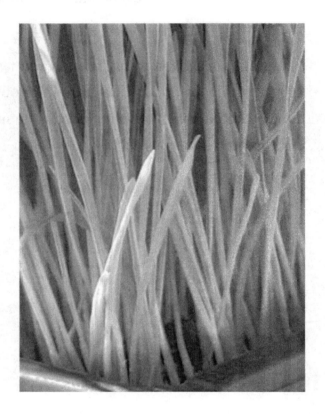

Wheatgrass juice is highly nutritious and beneficial because of the *synergy* of the absorbable contents in this complete food. A few included nutrients are:

- Magnesium
- Calcium
- Potassium
- Phosphorus
- Iron

- Selenium
- Chromium
- Zinc
- Chlorophyll
- Vitamins A, C, E, B-6, K, Folic acid
- Additional wide spectrum of minerals and trace elements
- Enzymes – like superoxide dismutase (SOD)
- Amino acids, Protein
- Additional powerful antioxidant enzymes

Imagine if Most People Truly Understood the Powerful Benefits of Wheatgrass Juice

As the global choir of wheatgrass juice lovers singing its praises grows in number, and as researchers continue to learn more about how this marvelous food can help both mankind and animals alike, the future looks bright for wheatgrass usage. Because of its great nutritional therapeutic qualities, I envision *all* hospitals, healing centers, and sports clubs around the world, one day providing access to freshly-squeezed wheatgrass juice.

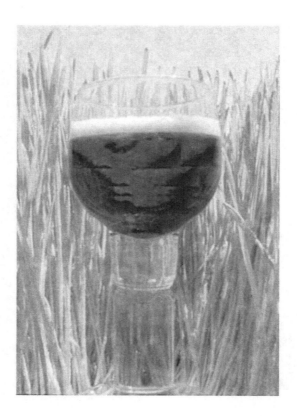

Can you imagine if wheatgrass juice was consistently "prescribed" to unwell people in nursing homes? I have *no doubt* that many of those with frail bodies would become better and more self-sufficient again.

Imagine wheatgrass juice being available in work place lunch rooms with the added benefit of more nourished employees. Your requests will help drive increased access to this juice. Imagine a day when anyone seeking to strengthen their health, increase their performance, overcome unwellness, help prevent illness, or "regain their groove," will immediately know to turn to wheatgrass juice for its valuable assistance!

Bodies and minds are *crying out* for more *raw* foods with health-building enzymes, plentiful minerals and trace elements—precisely what good wheatgrass juice offers. Once you start growing wheatgrass and drink its impressive juice and receive its "positive vibrations" regularly, you will notice increased vitality, and a sense of well-being.

"You have been guided to the richest nutritional liquid known to man in the chlorophyll-rich juice of wheatgrass. This substance, found in the blades of newly sprouting wheat, taken freshly-gathered and fed into the human digestive system each day, will add nutritive substances vital to health that have been removed or lost from many of the foods now obtainable, foods that are often not merely days, but weeks or months old."

—Dr. G.H. Earp-Thomas
World Expert on Grass and Soil Analyzation

Chapter 1: Wheatgrass Growing Preparation

Grow your way to better health!

How Should Healthy Wheatgrass Appear?

To begin, wheatgrass communicates its health to you through its color and visual liveliness. When in its peak state of health and maturity, it appears to be just begging you to consume it.

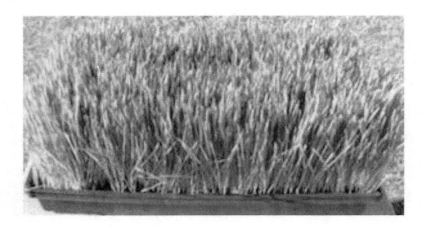

The health of the seed and soil and the nutrients taken in by the plant, affect the visual appearance of the blades of wheatgrass. Here are some good wheatgrass characteristics:

• Richer, darker green pigment is ideal—darker green is better

• Wider tipped blades of grass exuberantly reaching upwards for the sun

• Minimal to no mold

• No smell of grass or any particular scent—until you harvest and juice it

• Juicier or moistfull looking

As it ages and is beyond its prime state of nutrition, it begins to wilt and yellows in color. Based on its visual appearance, you will not be so inclined to consume it. If your wheatgrass is light green in color and looking withered, it is nutritionally inferior.

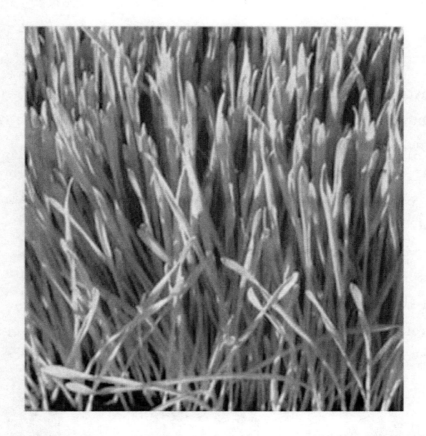

Wheatgrass is a true sunshine plant which *captures* the sun's electrical energy and creates fabulous chlorophyll— the plant's green blood which is actually quite similar to human blood. Take in its electrical vibrancy by juicing it in its peak state of vitality and then drink this wonderful blend of electrolytes.

Grow Barley Grass Too

Barley grass, which produces a slightly wider blade of grass, can be grown the *exact same* way as shown in this *How to Grow Glorious Wheatgrass at Home Tutorial*:

• I enjoy growing the barley grass too

• The taste is slightly more bitter

• Make sure you buy the *whole barley seed unhulled* (with the hull) or the barley seed won't sprout.

• Some claim barley grass is even more nutritious than the wheatgrass

• Wheatgrass is more popular, but I believe they are both exceptional

• You can grow them both to see which one you prefer

• You can even grow other cereal grasses like Kamut grass, rye grass, or spelt grass—once you obtain the seeds

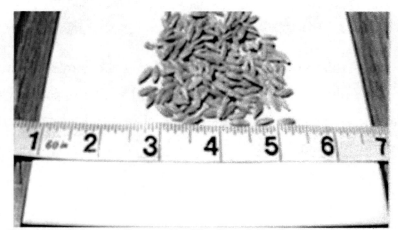

Barley seed must be unhulled, with the hull, to sprout.

So again, if you are a barley grass lover, just read through this *How to Grow Glorious Wheatgrass at Home Tutorial* and apply what you learn to grow your barley grass too.

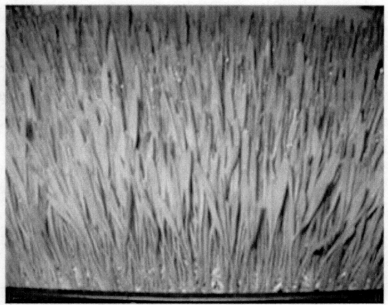

Barley grass grows equally well.

You will enjoy each of these fabulous raw, organic, green vegetables.

Wheatgrass Growing Supplies Checklist

Initially, when buying your wheatgrass growing supplies, buy them more conservatively. As you incorporate wheatgrass juice into your diet, and based upon your growing and consumption preferences, you can buy more seeds, soil, and trays accordingly. At the back of this tutorial, are excellent references for buying the key recommended growing supplies.

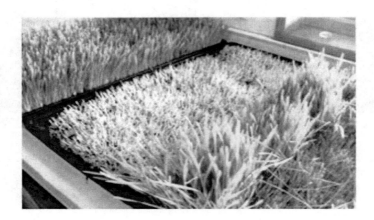

I am happy to share these simple and effective growing wheatgrass methods I have learned through much time and practice. But, of course you can use your own creativity too as there is not *one* exact right way to grow it. Below are the basic wheatgrass growing supplies you will need:

- Wheatgrass juicer
- Wheatgrass seeds – preferably organic
- Wheatgrass growing trays (12 - 15 ounces juice per tray)
- Bowl for soaking your seeds
- Colander – fine meshed
- Watering can with sprinkler head and/or pump sprayer container
- Good sludge-free top soil, or potting soil, or gardening soil, and/or optional compost
- Mineral rich and ocean based fertilizer – optional
- Soil sifter – optional
- 2-ounce shot glass for measuring juice

Ideal Wheatgrass Growing Temperature Range

Wheat seeds can actually germinate in soil temperatures from **40° - 99°** Fahrenheit. However optimally, indoor wheatgrass prefers to be grown in approximately **65° - 75°** Fahrenheit, but these temperatures *are not* essential for beautiful homegrown indoor wheatgrass. In the wintertime, place your growing trays in a warmer place.

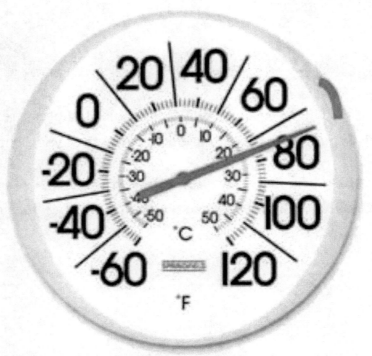

Optimal growing temperature is 65° - 75° F.

The healthier and stronger your wheat seed, the more it is nourished and supported, the greater its ability to better handle colder temperatures and warmer temperatures outside the 65° - 75° F range. Also, the healthier seeds will better withstand over watering or under watering conditions.

In other words*, healthier* and *well nourished* seeds are more resilient and do a far better job of handling stress—just like us. You will learn my favorite method for *increasing* the resiliency of your growing wheatgrass seeds, through sea solids (mineral rich sea salt) nourishment.

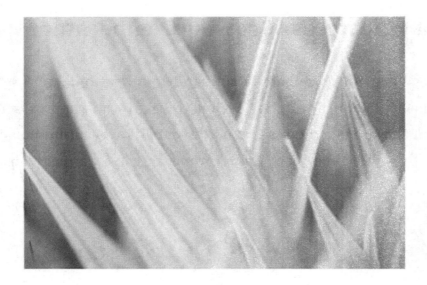

Warmer temperatures will speed up growth, and cooler temperatures outside the ideal growing range will slow down the germination and growth of your wheatgrass.

If growing temperature is greater than 80° F, you can increase air circulation to also counter the increased possibility of more mold. A ceiling fan or small portable circulating fan works well.

Determine Wheatgrass Tray Placement

You will first need to determine where you will place your indoor wheatgrass trays. I usually have two trays of wheatgrass growing on my kitchen counter. If growing more than a few trays, I also grow the wheatgrass on a table in my breakfast room.

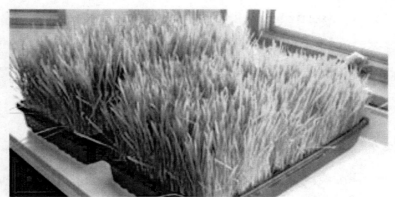

Wheatgrass is next to east facing window.

Start the second tray about midway through the full growing cycle of the first batch, so a fresh tray is always ready.

- Choose a location that offers lots of indirect sunlight
- Wheatgrass grows best indoors with indirect sunlight
- Wheatgrass does not need to be right next to a window to flourish
- During first few days of germination, no light is required
- Your seeds will be covered up for approximately 48 hours during the first few days of sprouting—to keep out any sunlight and promote quicker and better germination
- Wheatgrass can grow with overhead indoor full spectrum lighting, though I don't think anything can surpass Mother Nature and her lighting from the real sun

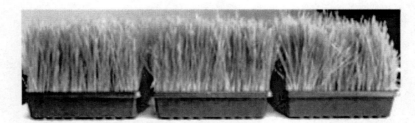

Wheatgrass flourishes 11 – 12 feet from kitchen window.

I place my wheatgrass trays to the left of my kitchen sink, below an east facing window. Sunlight shines in from the east in the morning. The back patio covering helps block the direct light. It receives the morning sunshine, more indirectly, until about 11:00 AM. Sometimes, I place my growing wheatgrass trays further away from the window.

> **"For the most part, I found that the chlorophyll extracted from sturdy, round-stemmed, shade-grown wheatgrass was softer, sweeter and had a more pleasant aroma than the flat leaf blade which fell limply to the ground under the direct rays of the summer's sun."**
> —*Ann Wigmore*

Either location, my wheatgrass turns out perfectly. Some place their wheatgrass trays in their utility rooms or basements. You will need to experiment to decide on the best location for you.

Wheatgrass Grows Well in Kitchen

There are many advantages to growing wheatgrass in your kitchen:

• Adds beautiful green color and emits oxygen into the air

• Wheatgrass is an excellent conversation piece. It's wonderful to be able to offer wheatgrass juice to your guests! Many times I deliver little paper Dixie cups with one to two ounces of freshly squeezed wheatgrass juice to my neighbors. It makes their day!

• Kitchens usually have nice indirect lighting

• You can set up your wheatgrass juicer right next to your wheatgrass tray (I attach my Hurricane Manual Juicer to my breadboard.)

• You can easily rinse off your wheatgrass before you juice it

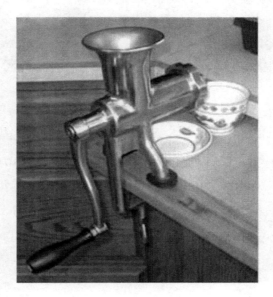

Additionally, the sink and quick access to water make the growing wheatgrass process easier:

• Kitchen faucet with spray nozzle can water wheatgrass

• Any excess water in bottom tray can be poured out into sink

Your consumption preference will determine the amount of wheatgrass trays you need to be growing at one time.

Wheatgrass Flourishes Inside or Outside

You can also place your wheatgrass tray in front of an open window and if there is a nice breeze, it can help with mold reduction. Additionally, many people also place the growing trays on benches, growing stands, or shelves—some choosing to build their own. Space, amount to be grown, and personal preference, will dictate your choice.

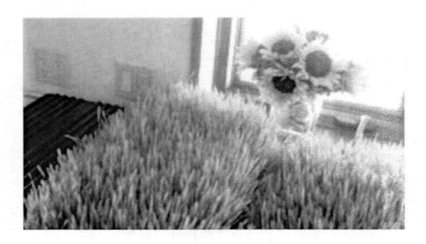

Sometimes, if the temperature outside is pleasant for wheatgrass growing, I will place my growing wheatgrass tray out on a stand or table in a *shaded* or *covered* area to avoid direct sunlight. Especially, if you have pets, above ground placement is better! Wheatgrass appreciates being placed outside in the elements and exposed to temperature vacillation, as it loves its *true* home and is accustomed to outside fluctuating conditions. You may notice the wheatgrass is even stronger, greener, and slightly sweeter tasting.

When outdoors, it has shown great resiliency in the colder and even freezing temperatures at night. Now, those wheat seeds will not be willing to sprout when too cool. However, as soon as the temperature rises, those little sprouts will too. Again, if placing wheatgrass trays outdoors in cooler temperatures, growth will be slower.

The ebb and flow of nature's wind and the outdoor habitat provide great mold reduction. However, birds do love to silently glide in and nibble on the little seeds. You'll need to trick the birds by occasionally changing the location of your trays—or place them in some sort of greenhouse, or cover them as shown.

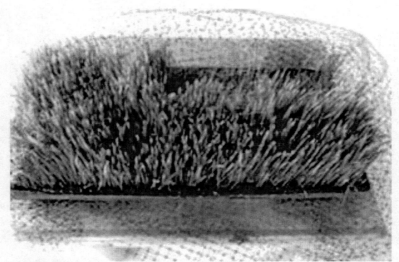

Double layer of BirdBlock Protective Mesh Covering is placed atop outdoor wheatgrass, kind of puffed up to allow grass to grow, keeps birds away. It can be tucked under tray.

"And Jesus sat beneath a gnarled and ancient tree, holding in his hands a small earthen pot; and in the pot was growing tender grass of wheat...

"And Jesus said, "Only when we chew well the blades of grass can the angel of Water enter our blood and give us strength. Eat, then, Sons of Light, of the most perfect herb from the table of our Earthly Mother, that your days may be long upon the earth, for such finds favor in the eyes of God."

—*Edmond Bordeaux Szekely*
The Essene Gospel of Peace (Book Four)

Chapter 2: How to Select Best Growing Seed

"In one sampling of 21 different samples of wheat seeds from around the world, there were 46,000 to 3,260,000 bacterial cells in one gram of wheat seeds."

—Gustafson and Parfeitt (1933)

Importance of Good Seed and Growing Conditions

Now, on to the seeds that are absolutely amazing *living* forms. Here you will learn why good wheatgrass or wheat seed selection matters.

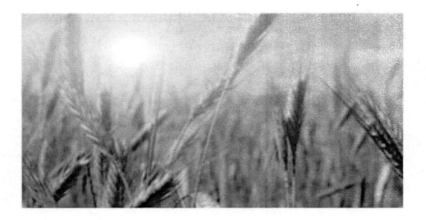

Each miraculous wheat seed contains an embryo—a baby wheat plant. *Individual* wheat seeds planted outdoors in the *right growing conditions* will first grow *one* blade of tender wheatgrass. This single grass blade will further develop to fulfill its destiny by becoming one strong, healthy, golden wheat plant. The wheatgrass stage is actually the beginning growth stage of the whole wheat plant. When the wheatgrass is young, it is especially nutritious.

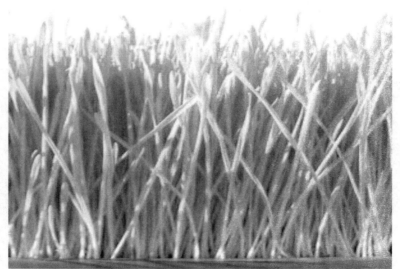

Good seed, with proper growing conditions, produces beautiful batches of wheatgrass.

The wheat plant, grown from just one grain or seed, will mature and produce its very own seeds (about 110) for harvesting. These produced wheat seeds are tiny new lives ready to begin the life-cycle of the wheat plant once more.

A well nourished mother wheat plant, that grew in good, healthy, non-toxic, nutrient rich soil and good growing conditions, will create *healthier* "offspring" seeds. These resulting desirable "offspring" seeds are more disease resistant and have a stronger immune system in place.

You want these healthier, good sprouting seeds. The better the condition of your wheatgrass seeds and the more optimal the growing conditions, the better your wheatgrass harvest will be.

Seed From a Healthy Soil Habitat is Best

The growing habitat of the mother wheat influences the microscopic biological world that is alive and well *even* on the *surface* of the seeds. The microbial communities on the surface of the seed vary according to its history.

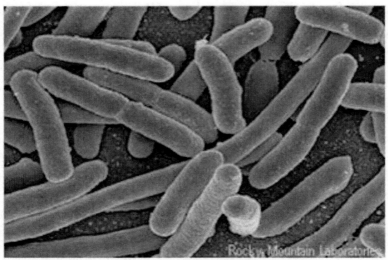
Bacteria exist on wheat seeds.

If the seeds came from a mother wheat plant that was grown in healthier soils abundant with beneficial miniscule life forms, organic matter, and a wide variety of minerals and trace elements, the pathogenic or unfriendly organisms will be held more in check. This means less of these undesirables will be negatively impacting the soil—thus healthier seeds.

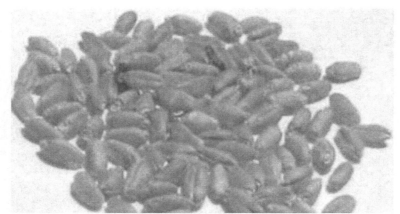
Healthy wheat seeds grow beautiful wheatgrass.

The "good guys" in the soil will be able to outcompete the "bad guys," like the pathogenic bacteria, for space and nutrients. Additionally, *good* soil bacteria thrive when minerals are readily available. Both friendly bacteria and bacterial pathogens found in the soil can actually become airborne and deposit themselves on the surface of wheat seeds that you later purchase. Microorganisms can actually exist *below* the surface of the seed too.

Yes, these minuscule life forms *truly live* in and on your seeds and communicate the health of the seeds—better bacteria, better seeds. You want the seeds that came from the best, least toxic, growing environment. This will help you understand just why the rinsing and presoaking of your seeds can greatly improve your success with growing wheatgrass.

Select Proper Growing Seeds

Again, listed are a few items that determine the seed pathogens, friendly bacterial flora, and also the overall health and immune system of the seed:

- Health of the mother wheat plant
- The growing environment of its mother plant
- Abundance and variety of minerals and trace elements, and amount of living beneficial micro and macro-organisms in the soil of its biological mother wheat plant
- Toxic chemicals applied to seed, soil, and mother wheat
- Storage and handling of seed
- Wheat variety

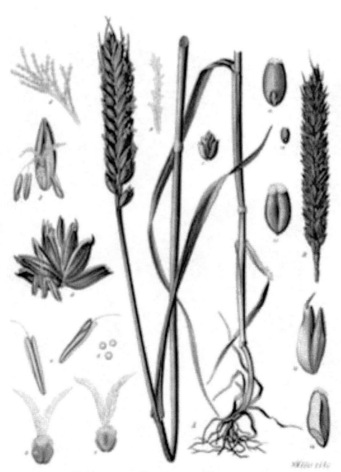

Triticum aestivum L. subsp. aestivum
Wheatgrass contains no gluten, unlike the wheat seed.

So, do obtain the best wheat seed you can for growing wheatgrass. Organic is the best, but it's not mandatory. And when selecting your wheat seed, understand wheat can be referred to by a few different names:

- Wheat seed
- Whole grain
- Wheat berry
- Wheat kernel
- Unrefined wheat grain

In this tutorial, I will usually use the term wheat seed.

Should I Choose Hard White or Hard Red Seed?

As mentioned, picking the right seed, from the best soil habitat, is a very important factor in successful wheatgrass growing. I recommend using the Hard White Seeds **or** Hard Red Wheat Seeds—*both* work equally well.

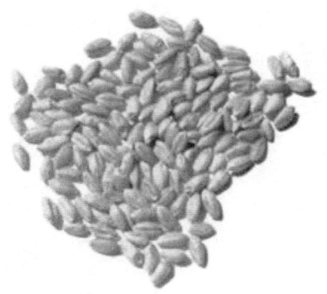

Hard white wheat seeds grow wheatgrass.

Hard White Seeds are small, long grains, with rich golden color:

- Make sure you *don't use* **Soft** Wheat Grains—they are not recommended for growing wheatgrass
- I especially like the Hard White Wheat
- I use the same Hard White Wheat to also make my delicious homemade bread recipe featured at HealthBanquet.com
- You can also buy wheat seed in bulk

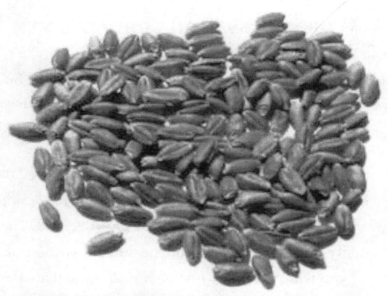

Hard red wheat seeds also grow wheatgrass.

Hard Red Wheat Seeds are darker, richer, and slightly reddish brown in color. You can *also* use these seeds for growing wheatgrass:

- Many wheatgrass seed suppliers will sell the Hard Red Wheat Seeds
- White *and* Red Wheat Seeds both produce *equally* nice wheatgrass
- Hard White Wheat Grains or Hard Red Wheat Grains are treated the same to grow wheatgrass

Wheatgrass Seed Comparison

As you can see, the Hard Red Wheat Seeds and Hard White Wheat Seeds are about the same size. You can experiment to discover which seed or grain *you* prefer for growing wheatgrass in your locale.

When growing your first batch of wheatgrass, I *highly* recommend buying the wheatgrass seeds mentioned in Chapter 13. Please buy your *first* supply of wheatgrass seeds from a supplier who sells *topnotch* wheatgrass growing seed. Then, after you have grown that high quality wheatgrass seed and personally witnessed your beautifully produced wheatgrass, you will now know *just how well* topnotch wheatgrass seeds will grow.

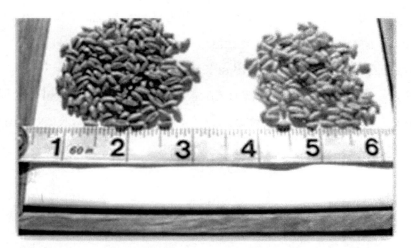

Hard red wheat versus hard white wheat—both grow excellent wheatgrass.

Later, if you purchase wheat seed *not* designated for wheatgrass growing, you can compare the wheatgrass growth from those seeds to the growth of the *original* wheatgrass seeds I recommend. In the future, purchase those seeds that are the highest quality, best price, easiest to access, and that grow the best wheatgrass for you. The less pesticides and unwanted chemicals on those seeds, the mother plant, and in the soil, the better off the seeds, us, and our environment.

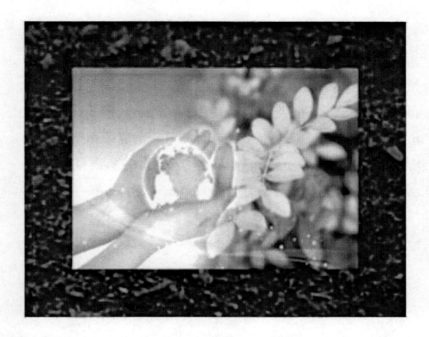

You may be able to find out if the growing soil is being replenished with a wide variety of minerals and trace elements. If possible and if not buying organic seeds, you can ask the seed distributor or grower if indeed they are using pesticides on the wheat—to help guide your buying decision.

Good Wheat Seed Characteristics

Again, seek higher quality seed:

- Fresher or more recently harvested seeds have a higher sprouting rate
- Wheat plants grown in mineral rich quality soil that is approved for organic production, or soil as close to that as possible, produce best seeds
- Preferably, seeds not fumigated and not treated with fungicides

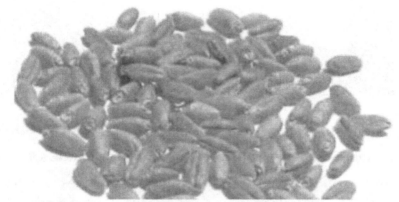

Favorable wheat seeds have a higher sprouting rate.

If you buy good sprouting wheat grains like I recommend, they should **maintain their germinating or sprouting ability for two years from harvest.** If the whole wheat grains are stored in a dry and cool location, they could last much longer.

Non-organic seeds coming from plants that have been heavily treated with herbicides, pesticides, fungicides, and synthetic fertilizers, are negatively impacted. **These harmful chemicals destroy the valuable friendly microscopic life in the soil—thus contributing to a seed with a weaker constitution and immune system.**

Favorable wheat seeds are fuller in appearance. They are the result of proper environmental conditions being met. Distressed grains, which are not graded for human consumption, appear small and shrunken.

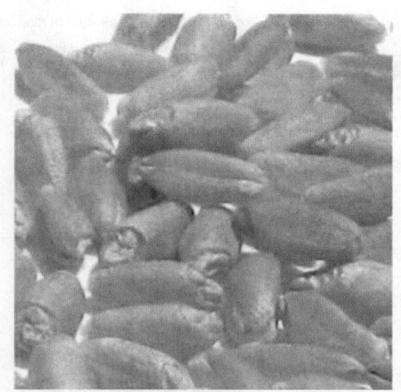

Favorable wheat seeds enlarged.

"A mere teaspoon of good garden soil, as measured by microbial geneticists, contains a billion invisible bacteria, several yards of equally invisible fungal hyphae, several thousand protozoa, and a few dozen nematodes."

—Jeff Lowenfels & Wayne Lewis
Teaming with Microbes

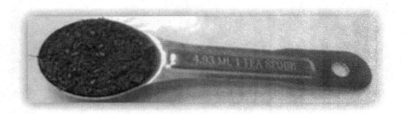

Chapter 3: How to Choose Good Soil and Avoid Unacceptable Soil

"Minerals from the soil nourish all creatures during their lives; and unto minerals of the soil all creatures ultimately return at their deaths....

"Healthy soil, good nutrition, and good health go hand in hand; and those creatures that contribute to the health of soils are obviously of the utmost importance for the well-being of the planet."

—James B. Nardi
Life in the Soil

The Soil—Grass—Animal Health Relationship is Important to Understand

The better the fertility or immune system of the precious growing soil, the better the immune system of the grass or plant, and therefore the better off the immune system of the animal or human from consuming this healthier grass or plant.

> **"When the pasture provides appropriate nutrition, veterinary bills—except for trauma—virtually disappear."**
> —*Charles Walters*

Poor grass will endure, but nutrient rich grass produces champions. **And animals can graze on stunningly beautiful grass and yet be in a starving situation because the visually misleading grass is actually deficient from its poverty stricken soil.**

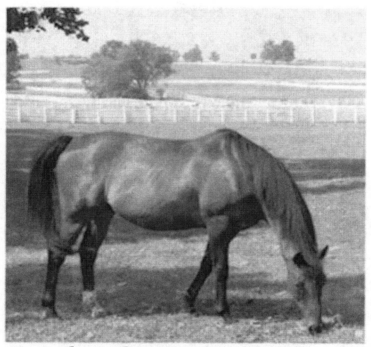

Race horses in Kentucky are known to be incredibly sturdy and fast from eating bluegrass from calcium rich soil—minerals pass from soil, to grass, to the horses.

Through consuming the wheatgrass juice, we are taking in its inherent resilience, hardy constitution, and powerful nutrition. The wider the selection of absorbable nutrients in the soil, the more nutrients there will be in our consumed wheatgrass from that soil.

> **"Both the human immune system and the plant immune system are *fundamentally* interdependent on the quality and fertility of the soil.**
>
> **"Our immune system, and *even our physical structure*, are a reflection of the foods we have eaten from either toxic and nutrient depleted soils, or wonderfully fertile soils."**

Plants, Animals, and Humans Are a Reflection of the Soil Quality

Healthier soils *help control diseases* within the soil, on the plants themselves, and also on the plant "offspring"—the seeds. This beneficial microbial population in the soil, both nourishes and protects the growing plant. The good "commando" bacteria are at the front line of defense within your soil. These natural defenses and nutrients within the soil contribute to a better environment for your wheatgrass seeds to dig in their roots to seek out nourishment, and grow into splendid blades of grass.

> **"On grass and forage that contains suitable fertility loads, the bovine's instincts will see to a diet that triggers hormone and enzyme systems capable of warding off viral, bacterial, fungal and even insect attacks."**
> —*Charles Walters*

This magnificent soil life actually produces soil nutrients and helps the plants to better assimilate the nutrients. Both the larger and microscopic organisms that contribute to the health of soils are clearly critical to the well-being of plant, animal, and human. **Healthy mineral rich soil, good foods from that soil, and good health are *intimately* related.**

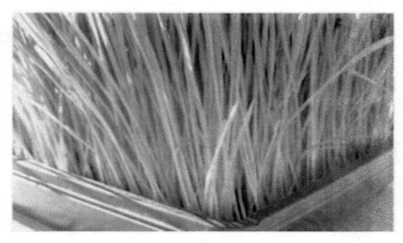

The condition of the soil and its ability to provide a continual supply of essential minerals will affect the health of the plant. Nutrients applied by foliar feeding will also influence the vigor of the plant.

Mother Earth's good soil nourishes and supports germinating seeds so they can better withstand environmental stresses. With an optimum growing environment including plentiful assimilable minerals, the growing wheatgrass can now focus more of its energies on fulfilling its mission of bringing forth vigorous, nutrient rich blades of grass.

Good Soil Characteristics for Wheatgrass Growing

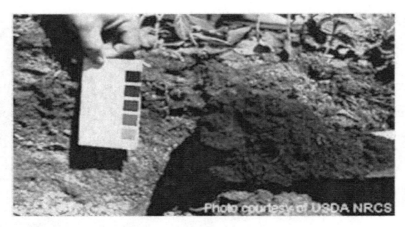

You want to obtain good soil for growing wheatgrass:

- Dark brown to black coffee-colored
- Rich in organic matter
- Smells earthy, fresh, and good—**it should not smell bad or offensive in any way**
- Able to hold water, yet still drains when too much exists
- Well aerated—light, airy, and porous allowing for good air circulation for biological activity, and space for soil biology to live
- Peat moss, vermiculite, or perlite work well
- Preferably, no herbicides, pesticides, chemical fertilizers, derivatives from sewage sludge, contaminants, animal or human manures (worm castings are fine)
- Full of a wide variety of minerals and trace elements

> **"Soil biology conserves fertility, and any 'fertilizer' that kills off soil biology does not deserve to be called a fertilizer."**
> —*Charles Walters*

On average, plants extract about 40 elements from the soil—*only if they exist in the soil.* **Most commercial fertilizers add a *maximum* of six minerals back to the soil which can be inadequate and create imbalances.**

If the minerals and elements are all supplied in the soil, the plant will be able to extract what it needs. If they are absent from the soil, the plant will be unable to absorb that particular mineral or element. Because of the high mineral extraction capability of wheatgrass, you would optimally like to make sure a *full* variety of these minerals and trace elements are in the soil.

Poor Soil Characteristics

Poor soil has unfavorable characteristics:

- Pale, compacted, mineral depleted
- Drains too well, won't retain any water, can smell bad
- Holds too much water becoming perhaps anaerobic with little air circulation
- Deficient in micro-organisms and macro-organisms
- Can contain contaminants if originating from sewage sludge

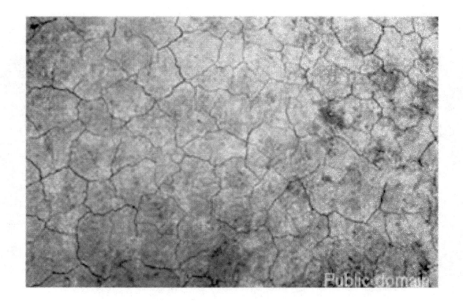

A plant grown in poor soil, *may* look healthy and taste OK, but it can still be nutrient deficient and missing valuable minerals it would have liked to absorb if they were in the soil.

> **"You can trace every sickness, every disease, and every ailment to a mineral deficiency."**
> —*Linus Pauling, MD*

Plants can also take in nutrients through their leaves (foliar applied). **Plants *cannot* create minerals, they must absorb them.** A *wide* variety of minerals, even if only available in minuscule amounts, are *essential* to the proper functioning of man. *Indeed* *in time*, more will be learned on how all the minerals in the atomic table benefit man on some level.

To ensure my soil has a *wide* collection of *easily absorbable* minerals, especially since the wheatgrass growing time frame is so short, I prefer adding mineral rich sea solids. The sea solids contain a huge array of minerals and trace elements that are consistently and *perfectly* proportioned by Mother Nature herself. You will learn about the sea solids in Chapter 5.

Superior Mineral and Trace Element Uptake
by Wheatgrass

Wheatgrass is superior when it comes to being able to extract nutrients from the soil. It has been known to absorb up to 90 elements plus. *If the elements are first in the soil, then wheatgrass can absorb them.* Truly extraordinary! Could its amazing element extraction abilities and the abundance of elements transferred into the wheatgrass be largely responsible for the powerful nutritional benefits one receives?

Unprocessed SEA-90 sea solids fertilizer contains 90 plus minerals and trace elements. More minerals continue to be discovered.

In *Fertility from the Ocean Deep*, by Charles Walters, he shares how when sea solids fertilizer is used, there is amazing mineral absorption from tomatoes (56), sweet potatoes (70), and the phenomenal wheatgrass (90) as you can see in the following chart. By fertilizing with the sea solids and water solution which I will explain later, the wheatgrass can *instantly* absorb all the elements it wants, so it can achieve its full genetic potential.

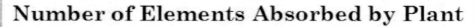

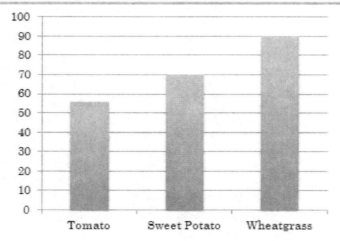

Which Soil or Soil Mixture Do I Use?

"Soil" seems to have very broad definitions. Additionally, there are so many names for bagged "soils" these days. Let's see, to name a few: Potting soil, gardening soil, planting mix, gardening mix, top soil, compost, peat moss. And just which bagged soil or soil mixture is most appropriate for wheatgrass growing?

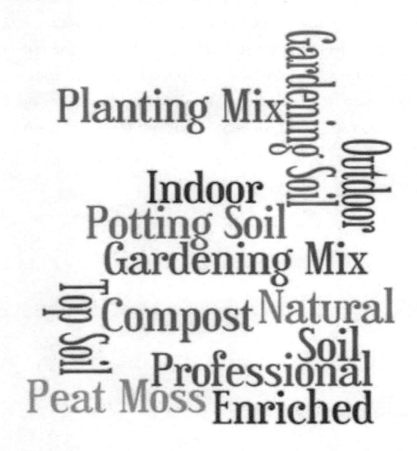

Each of these different bags of soil and soil blends have different ingredients sourced from different materials and locations. They also may contain different kinds of fertilizers. Read the microscopic label to better understand all that is found inside.

Alright, if purchasing your soil, how can you choose real high quality soil, and what is the best soil blend combination? No worries, I will provide guidance when you read on. Also, are you wondering if there are "soils" that should be avoided? Absolutely, and I will shortly get into that too.

> "Dr. William Albrecht of the Department of Agriculture at the University of Missouri used to say, 'Disease preys on an undernourished plant.' I say, 'Disease preys on an undernourished body.'"
> —Dr. Bernard Jensen

Please note, if you have access to good growing soil in your backyard or from another well-known connection, feel free to use it. If purchasing soil, the following advice will help guide you to a better soil choice. It will also teach you to do your homework before you use any "free" compost that may be given away without knowing just where that compost originated from and what could be hiding inside.

What Kind of Soil Does Wheatgrass Prefer?

Once you know which soils to avoid and some good soil choices you can make, you can have fun experimenting with different soil blends—you can even make your own soil blends.

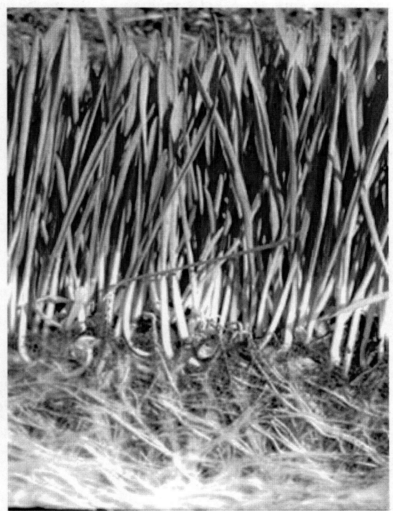

Microorganisms in the soil feast and multiply on SEA-90 sea mineral solids and water fertilizing solution.

And don't worry, there really is not *one perfect* soil blend "recipe" for planting your wheat seeds. **When it comes to growing it, wheatgrass is quite easy to please**.

> **"*Basically*, the wheatgrass wants a nice nutrient rich growing soil. It wants a growing environment where it can easily shoot forth its roots to absorb food, where air can freely circulate, and where water is nicely retained, yet not soggy, and drains nicely."**

Wheatgrass is a remarkable superfood. But keep in mind, the more *readily absorbable* minerals and trace elements in the soil, the better *fed* your wheatgrass. Hence, the better *fed* you will be when you drink this emerald green wonder which is like a "stream of life."

Let's first go over a few "soil" definitions....

Definitions of Different Kinds of Growing Mediums

Soil - A combination of rock broken into small particles, decaying organic matter, and *fully* decayed matter (humus). Different rock contains different blends of minerals and trace elements. Soil may also contain living organisms, micro and macro-sized. Soil varies from location to location depending on specific rocks that have been broken down and made their way into it. Also, organic matter and its nutrient and mineral profile can vary, thus affecting the soil ingredients.

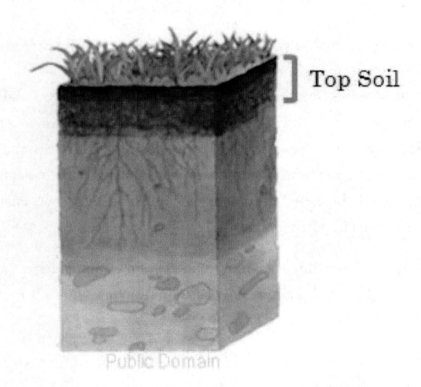

Top Soil – Layer of soil closest to the surface and it usually has more organic matter, or *fully* decomposed matter.

Potting Soil – It usually is made up of peat moss, shredded bark and vermiculite or perlite, plus other added non-soil ingredients. Technically, it is not real soil in that it is lacking in fractionated pieces of rocks with their minerals. It contains little to no soil or dirt. Potting soil is therefore very lightweight, is basically sterile, and contains little nutrients.

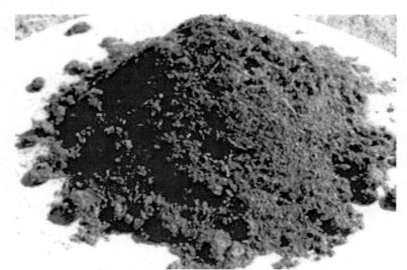

Sphagnum peat moss holds water and air, but it is not a source of nutrients for wheatgrass.

Sphagnum Peat Moss – *Decayed* more compact Sphagnum moss is called Sphagnum peat or Sphagnum peat moss. It is a common ingredient in soil-less mixes because it is widely available, relatively inexpensive, and has desirable physical characteristics. It holds a lot of water and air, and decomposes very slowly. Since peat is quite acidic, limestone can optionally be added to the mix to help balance the pH. Peat moss is *not* a source of plant nutrients in potting mixes.

Humus – Stable, long-lasting residual made from *completely* decayed material. Humus is a fraction of the soil matter that assists in making minerals available to plant rootlets.

Compost – Plant food from organic matter that has decayed and which can now be used as fertilizer for your wheatgrass. It looks like dark brown crumbles. It contains micro-organic nutrients plus desirable bacteria and organisms. Its mineral composition varies according to the minerals that were in the *original* non-decayed matter.

Fertilizer – Plant food which can be either organic (composed of organic matter, plant or animal), or inorganic (composed of synthetic chemicals and or minerals). The better and wider variety of food available, the better nourished your wheatgrass will be.

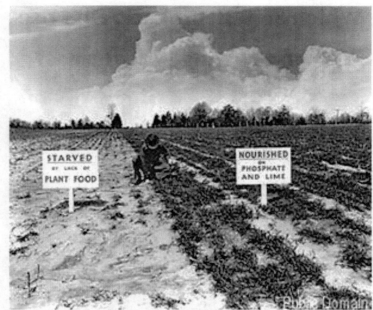

Fertilizers encourage growth as shown in test.

Worm Castings – Nourishing plant food, also known as vermicompost or vermicastings, created when organic matter passes through the digestive tract of earthworms and is excreted. It is 100% organic and natural earthworm manure brimful of beneficial bacteria and fungi. The earthworm's extraordinary digestive system process transforms its consumed matter into a fantastic fertilizer supplement that the plants absolutely love. Plus, it is 100% safe around children and pets. This worm manure is *marvelous* for wheatgrass growing.

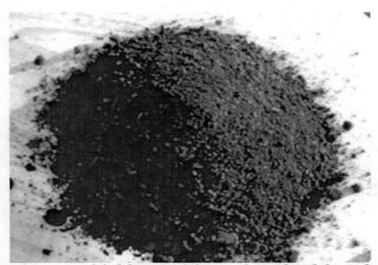

Worm castings are highly nutritious plant food for wheatgrass.

Which Soil Blend Ratio Do I Use
When Growing Wheatgrass?

I like to experiment with my growing wheatgrass "soils." When purchasing "soils" (top soil, gardening soils, compost, peat moss, worm castings, etc.), I prefer the highest quality I can find.

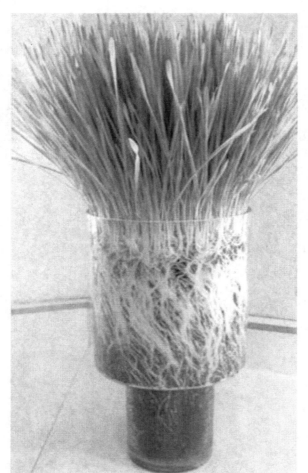

Extensive root system is seeking and transferring water and nutrients to growing wheatgrass blades.

Your personal observations and growing success will guide you in your growing medium choices. Here are a few soil blends with which I have had success:

- 100% top soil
- 50% top soil and 50% compost

- 25% Peat moss and 75% compost
- 100% compost (Compost can be more expensive or more work for you to make at home, so you can use it more sparingly by diluting with other soils.)
- 90% peat moss or potting mix, and 10% worm castings
- Fertilize with sea solids ocean minerals—my favorite full selection of minerals fertilizer (If I grow wheatgrass with compost or worms castings, I still use beneficial sea solids.)

So go ahead and have fun, and experiment. Feel free to come up with your own soil blends and ratios for the roots of your wheatgrass to proliferate. It is *perfectly fine* to vary your soil blends. Through variation and differing blend ratios, you will be planting in soils with slightly different nutriment profiles.

How Can I Choose a High Quality Soil?

Here are some ideas to find *high quality* soil and to avoid the many deceiving and rebranded soil products derived from sewage sludge that are commonly available today. **You *do not* want soil products made from sewage sludge.**

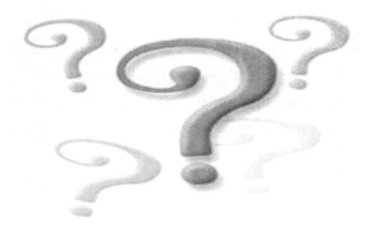

1. Ask questions when shopping for soil or soil amendment products. Shop where the staff is well informed and can honestly and intelligently answer your questions.

2. Contact the manufacturer and distributor. Trustworthy companies will provide laboratory results and other data about where they obtain the material for their products.

3. Use soil amendment products approved for certified organic crop production. The Organic Materials Review Institute is a non-profit organization that determines which input products are allowed for use in organic production and processing.

Choosing soil products with the below OMRI Listed® Seal on the soil label or bag ensures the soil is not made from sewage sludge.

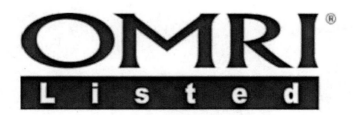

You can access the lists of soil and soil amendment products given the outstanding OMRI approval at www.omri.org. The OMRI Products List is the most complete directory of products for organic production or processing. You will love the companies and products you discover. The OMRI Listed® Seal assures you the product has passed OMRI expert review for use in organic production.

Good Soil Matters

Again, when buying soil or soil amendments, including compost, you do not want it to be derived from toxic sewage sludge. The OMRI Listed® Seal assures you the soil product is not made from sewage sludge—unwanted sewage sludge products are not allowed in organic foods production.

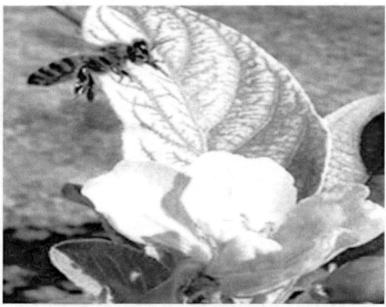

Just as a bee zeros in on quality nectar to nourish itself, you are to zero in on quality soil to better nourish your wheatgrass.

You may find *what appears to be* a high quality soil product that does not have the OMRI Listed® Seal. Before you buy it, just ask the manufacturer or knowledgeable retailer to make sure it is not made from sewage sludge.

Once you have found high quality growing mediums, you will enjoy continually experimenting with them. Over time though, you may settle in on a few wheatgrass growing soil blend "recipes," based on the resources you have access to and the success you have.

Each soil habitat and its mineral composition is a little different. Each soil can vary physically, chemically, and biologically. Healthy soil variety is a good thing. I cannot imagine there being any two *"identical* in composition" soils.

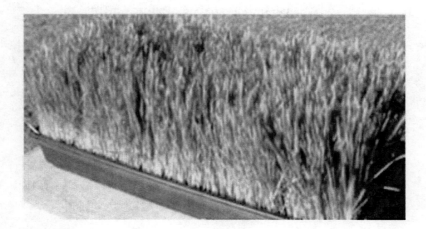

When experimenting with your selected soil mixtures, observe how your wheatgrass grows with them, and notice the color of the grass leaves. Pay attention to its level of vitality. You want "happy looking," perky, vigorous, vibrant green wheatgrass.

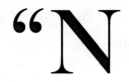"Not yet, however, have we recognized soil fertility as the food producing forces within the soil that reveal national and international patterns of weakness and strength."

—*Dr. Weston A. Price*
Nutrition and Physical Degeneration

Chapter 4: If Using Compost, Choose Carefully

"No civilization has ever lived beyond the health of its soil, and only by the most artificial means have we stretched this rule and extended this civilization."

—*Dr. Bernard Jensen & Mark Anderson*
Empty Harvest

Composted Manure Not Recommended For At Home Wheatgrass Growing

Ann Wigmore was a big advocate of adding compost to her soil when growing wheatgrass—to add further nutrients to it. You can absolutely use compost for your wheatgrass growing too, but you don't *have* to. If your compost contains larger particles that interfere with your wheatgrass growing, you can easily make a soil sifter to filter them out. I show you how to make a soil sifter in Chapter 10.

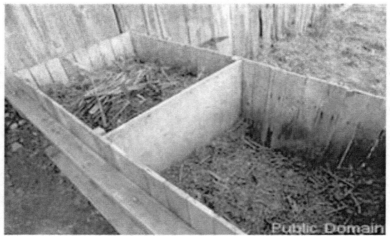

Composting Container

Ann Wigmore did *not* recommend compost made from animal manure for wheatgrass growing at home, as it can still contain harmful bacteria even after composted.

Naturally, *fully* mature compost made from the manure of *healthy* animals (that is not contaminated from antibiotics, pesticides, herbicides, or growth hormones) is *highly* valuable in agriculture, *however,* for wheatgrass growing at home, you can err on the side of caution and not use compost sourced from manure.

Some companies that sell soil and compost are *manure free* and state *No Poop* on the soil or compost bag—which makes it real clear there is no manure. You can see this *No Poop* labeling on the bag shown.

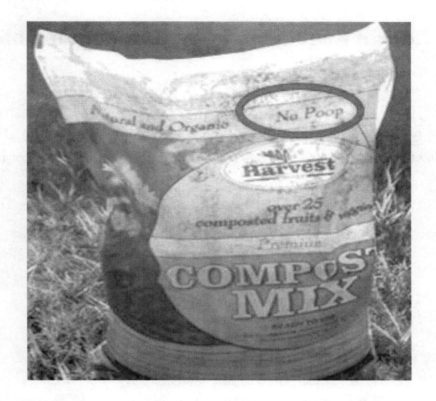

Have I ever grown my wheatgrass in soils with manure in the past? Yes, I have—with chicken manure and/or bat guano. However, I now do my best to avoid manure for my wheatgrass growing.

Guidelines if Regularly Using Homemade Compost for Wheatgrass Growing

Ann Wigmore exchanged her continuously recycled compost every few years to make sure the compost stayed properly balanced. I think that is a good idea. Let me explain.

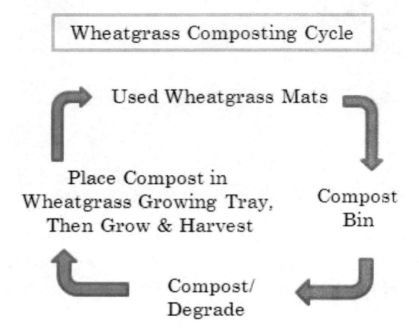

Wheatgrass Composting Cycle

Used Wheatgrass Mats

Place Compost in Wheatgrass Growing Tray, Then Grow & Harvest

Compost Bin

Compost/ Degrade

Basically, if you compost at home, you can grow your wheatgrass using your homemade compost. After harvesting your wheatgrass, take the used and clipped wheatgrass mat and put it into your compost bin to decompose. Once the spent mat is converted back to compost, you can use that new batch of compost again in your growing tray for your next batch of wheatgrass.

However, after a year or two of this recycling cycle, the compost could become out of balance. It has been awhile since that recycled compost has been exposed to nature's elements—sun, rain, air, and wind. Nature's elements help to keep the soil in balance and healthier. To *rebalance* this compost, you can place that compost in the soil in your yard and expose it to the seasons and its natural environment again.

> **"Life behaviors are more closely linked with soils as the basis of nutrition than is commonly recognized."**
> —*Dr. Weston A. Price*

Another idea is to give your compost to a small farmer, or a friend who needs it for their yard or garden. And hopefully, they have some outdoor, element-exposed compost they would trade you. Then begin the usage of the new compost for a year or two—until it is time to rebalance it in the outdoors once again.

Compost is a Valuable Natural Fertilizer

Good quality compost is a wonderful natural fertilizer:

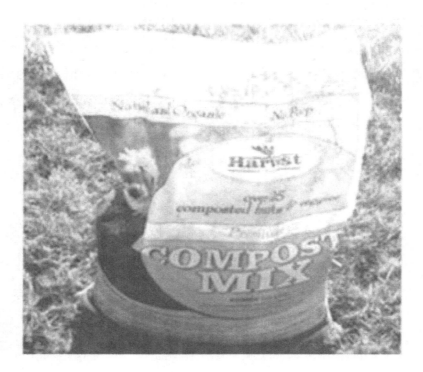

- Increases soil aeration
- Enhances soil structure
- Boosts ability of plant to uptake soil nutrients
- Increases capacity of soil to hold moisture
- Adds a wealth of beneficial biological life forms and a huge variety of plant nutrients

To repeat, if you choose to use compost, you can use **50% soil to 50% compost**. Otherwise, you can select a ratio of compost to soil, based on what works best for you.

You can make your own compost or buy compost. Buying compost is easier, but it is more expensive and requires some research on your part. Remember, you can also look for the OMRI Listed® Seal on your purchased compost bag to make sure it is not made from potentially dangerous sewage sludge.

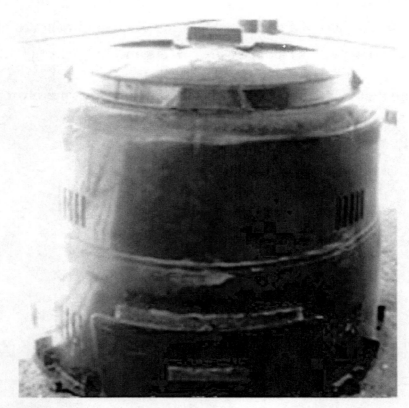

I obtained this free black compost bin from the Public Works Department in my town.

Contact your local city or town government, or solid waste utility to find out if they offer free, or greatly reduced in price, compost bins. They may even offer workshops on composting.

"I have used these sea solids as plant food in experiments to prove that these elements in perfect balance will grow chemically perfect plants.

"Note that I did not try to synthesize anything, but merely took what nature already offered."

—Maynard Murray, M.D.
Sea Energy Agriculture

Chapter 5: My Favorite Highly Effective Fertilizer, How to Use, and Why it's Fabulous

"All truth passes through three stages. First, it is ridiculed. Second, it is violently opposed. Third, it is accepted as being self-evident."

—*Arthur Schopenhauer*

Sea Solids are Abundantly Available to Remineralize and Refertilize our Depleted Soils

Properly harvested sea solids (crystal-like mineral salts remaining after water is evaporated from seawater) that capture the wonderful essence of the sea itself, are a fantastic, *highly effective,* and convenient fertilizer for growing wheatgrass. Please keep in mind, Ann Wigmore was able to overcome gangrene and avoid leg amputations largely by eating the grass right off the ground. So please don't worry *too* much if you have the *perfect* soil for your wheatgrass. But *do realize,* better soil *absolutely* equals better wheatgrass. And if you are going to take the time to grow precious wheatgrass, it is highly advantageous to optimize its nutritional qualities.

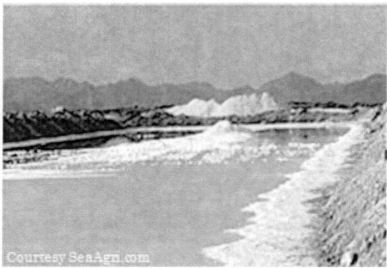

Wheatgrass loves the seawater-like quality of salty sea solids mixed with water.

I started experimenting with sea salt usage for wheatgrass growing, as I knew of the powerful anti-bacterial properties and nutrients in *unprocessed* sea salt. Initially, I was just hoping it would assist in mold reduction—which it did. However, by incorporating sea salt into my wheatgrass growing, I was *also* both surprised and captivated when I saw my wheatgrass sprouts reaching upward with an *increased* level of vigor.

Clearly understanding the positive value of using *whole* sea salt for my wheatgrass growing, I experimented to find the best performing "sea salt." When it comes to sea salt, there is a *huge variety* in quality, and you want the best. I will share my favorite ocean based "sea salt" fertilizer with you.

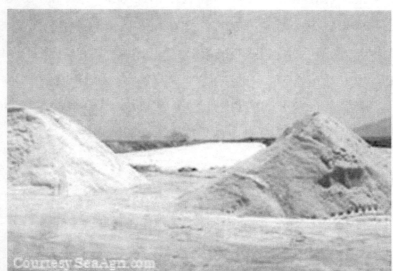

Harvested SEA-90 sea solids are available at SeaAgri-com.

My favorite "sea salt" for wheatgrass growing is actually *accurately* referred to as "SEA-90 sea solids." They are produced through *sun* drying from the ocean, and include the *entire* mineral, trace element, and biological package.

Wheatgrass Thrives with Salty Mineral Solution at Right Salinity Level

Believe it or not, wheatgrass and other plants, *love* salty sea solid minerals from the ocean, when water is added to them. The *secret,* is to make sure the salt solution is at the right salinity level for that particular plant. Plants cannot absorb elements from the soil unless they are in *liquid* form—and sea solids are *100%* soluble (*fully* liquefying and dissolving when water is mixed with them) and are available for *immediate* plant uptake—*perfect* for the short growing time frame of wheatgrass.

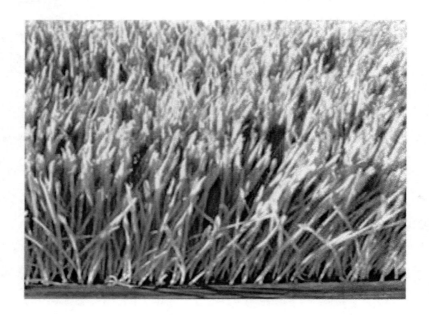

Non-refined SEA-90 sea solids are simple to use, affordable, sustainable, earth-friendly, easy to store, and a *highly productive* way to provide a complete assortment of elements to the happily absorbing grass. Later, when you are fortunate to drink this juice from the wheatgrass, you will take in its bounty of replenishing nutrients.

It is indeed fact that the naturally proportioned, perfectly balanced chemistry of minerals and trace elements found in the ocean solids themselves, are not only clearly optimal for the growth and nourishment of sea vegetation and other sea life but *also* for land life—including vegetation, humans, animals, and of course wheatgrass. I explain how to make this excellent fertilizing agent in Chapter 5.

> **In 1865, Johan Georg Forchhammer found that regardless of variation in salinity, the ratio of major salts in samples of seawater from locations around the world, was constant. (Excess minerals fall to the bottom of the ocean.) This constant ratio of ocean elements is known as the Principle of Constant Proportions.**

Using the recommended SEA-90 sea solids as a safe and natural fertilizer, and understanding the wide amount of nutrients the wheatgrass can absorb from it, is a very satisfying feeling. **Again, when sea solids are combined with water, and thus dissolved, their elements are *instantly* available for wheatgrass uptake.** Let's learn more about why this unheralded, good for land life, salty fertilizer is so beneficial....

How Can We be Blinded to the Fertility Gifts of the Ocean for Agriculture?

First, here is a little fun science to help you understand our interconnectedness with sea salt, and to appreciate the value of sea mineral solids as a fertilizer for your wheatgrass growing.

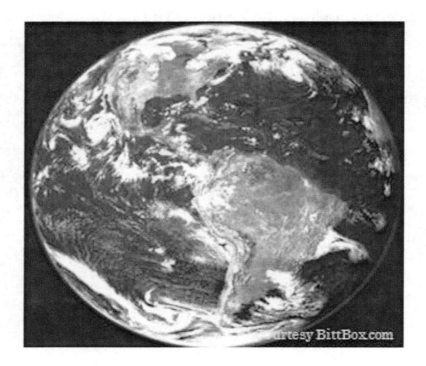

Scientists believe liquid water began accumulating on the surface of the Earth about 4 billion years ago, forming the early ocean. There is evidence of microscopic life later in the seas about 3.4 billion years ago, with other bigger life forms evolving from the ocean to the land millions of years ago.

The ancient salty seas covered *most* of the surface of the Earth, exposing very little land. These ancient salty seas were believed to be even saltier than the oceans of today. Estimates of the salinity range of the early oceans was between 1.2 to 2 times our present day average ocean salinity levels.

Salt Content of Seawater VS Human Blood	
Sea Water	**Human Blood**
Appx. 3.5%	Appx. 1% (0.9)
The body contains the 0.9% salty "sea water" within its internal fluids: tears, saliva, sweat, amniotic fluid, cell cytoplasm, etc.	

Today, our oceans are an average of 35 salinity which means 35 pounds of salt per 1,000 pounds of sea water—about 3.5% salt. Human blood contains about 0.9 percent salt—almost 1% salt.

Also now, about 71% of the earth is covered by oceans well seasoned with salt. About 80 percent of all life on Earth is found in the salty, life-sustaining oceans. Estimations indicate if the abundant salt in the oceans could be removed and spread evenly over the Earth's land surface, it would form a layer more than 500 feet (166 meters) thick. Plenty of salt to be used for your wheatgrass growing!

The Secret to Sea Minerals as an Effective Fertilizer is the Right Salinity Level

Different plants prefer different salinity levels in the soil. In agriculture, too high a degree of salinization interferes with the growth of all but those plants specifically adapted for it. On the other hand, with the right amount of salinity, many plants can *absolutely* flourish.

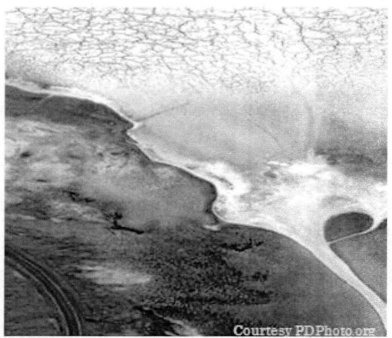

Too high a concentration of sea salt and crops won't grow.

After natural catastrophes like tsunamis, widespread crop damage can occur from the onslaught of ocean salt. However, some farmers have been happily surprised to learn the recovery of the soil (the right salinity level from later dispersed and rain-diluted ocean salt) allowed for new crops to successfully grow again—in a far shorter time than anticipated. In fact, after the 2004 tsunami in Indonesia, they found the salty fertilizer *doubled* their rice yield and other crops truly thrived.

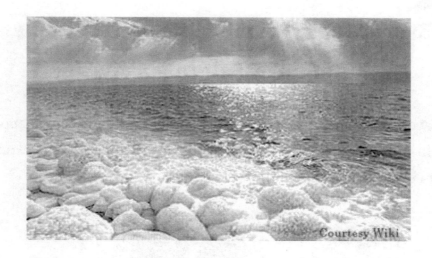

Courtesy Wiki

The full variety of oceanic elements are *perfectly* balanced and have not been manipulated by man. The humans and animals eating foods that have been fertilized with this "full essence from the ocean," *tremendously benefit.*

In Japan after the ravaging 2011 tsunami, farmers found the salty soil to be *ideal* for growing cotton. When crops are fertilized with a *full* spectrum of sea minerals that represent the "heart of the ocean," it is surprisingly discovered that a wide variety of plants do *exceptionally* well and produce mineral rich crops that have *increased resistance* to disease. Abundant and dissolvable sea minerals are excellent for wheatgrass, and fortunately sea mineral farming is gaining momentum for an improved tomorrow.

Every Single Form of Life on Our Planet
Requires Salt to Survive

Salt beds or deposits on land resulted from evaporated ancient seas—trapped when land masses arose from the oceans. When the ocean water evaporates, the elements solidify. This *unprocessed* sea salt contains all the elements supporting life.

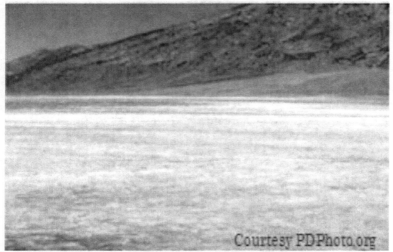

Dried salt beds remain from evaporated ancient seas.

The needed "ingredients" for the ocean to *precisely* make its health promoting saline "soup" come from different sources:

• Over the believed billions of years, eroded mineral rocks, mountains, and the Earth's crust have been transported to the sea from rains and streams

• Gaseous components released from the Earth's crust through volcanic openings or that came from the atmosphere

• Superheated water, rich with dissolved minerals gushing through hydrothermal vents in the bottom of the oceans

• Volcanoes erupting hot rock under the ocean which dissolves

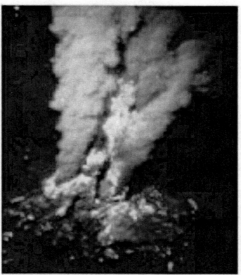

Hydrothermal vent discharges mineral rich water, and bacteria flourish around these vents.

Salt is the only rock eaten by human beings. It is an instrumental source of nutrients needed for the very survival of humans and animals—that need more salt than people. In fact, many formerly created roads were simply widened trails that were originally created by animals in search of salt licks. Villages were started at the end of such trails where salt was found, to have a close supply of their *essential for living* salt.

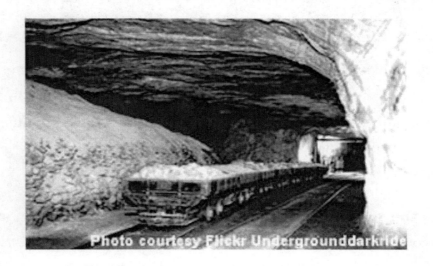

Photo courtesy Flickr Undergrounddarkride

In every century, on each continent, the predominant people were the ones that were in control of the potentially lucrative salt trade. Many *extremely powerful* salt empires were built.

We Carry the "Sea" Within Us
Non-Refined Sea Salt is Our Friend

A healthy adult body contains about 250 grams of salt. This amount would fill three salt shakers. Since our bodies continually lose salt through our functions and activities, the lost salt supply needs to be continually replaced. Salt is necessary for the delivery of nutrients, the transmitting of nerve impulses, and the contractions of the heart and other muscles. Sea salt elements promote respiratory health, blood sugar health, sinus health, bone strength, plus so much more.

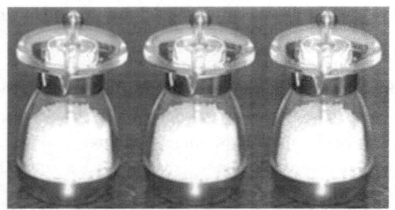

On average, there are three salt shakers worth of salt in each adult.

Additionally, scientists believe all plant cells evolved from ancient salty oceans. Surviving and flourishing in such a briny environment dates back to these earliest plants. Understanding how indispensible unrefined sea salt is to *living* organisms should help us *easily* understand the incredible value it can play in agriculture, gardening, and wheatgrass growing.

Importantly, the sea denizens *perfectly* sustained in the pure ocean are *not* sustained from water and *refined* salt. They are nourished from *non*-refined sea salt containing a *complete* medley of trace minerals and elements in *rightly balanced* proportions, the way Mother Nature orchestrates.

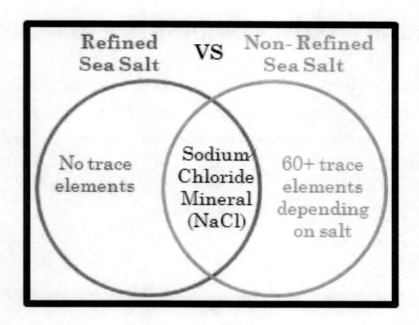

The SEA-90 sea solids are not processed and stripped of any key minerals and trace elements. They consist of the *balanced* and *entire* mineral health banquet of the nourishing sea, minus the water—a mixture of 90 plus minerals and trace elements. *Delightfully* and *factually*, wheatgrass grows quite well in a higher saline environment.

Wheat Plant Flourishes With Sea Solids Fertilization

SEA-90 sea solids fertilization can support the wheat plant on land—the very wheat plant that so generously supplies the wheat seeds for growing young wheatgrass. Beneficial microbes feast on the sea solids and then increase in population, *further* enriching the soil.

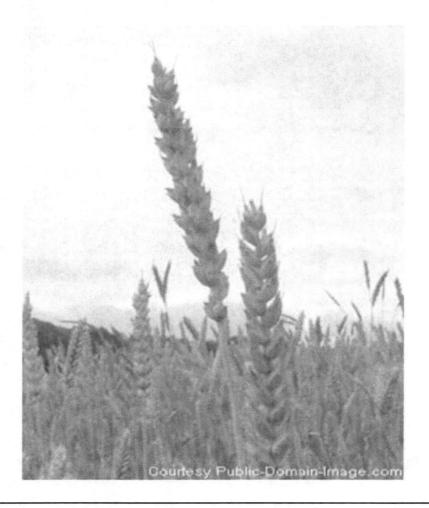

"All the problems inherent in our modern system can be eliminated with the application of Sea Energy in Agriculture and good sense in Processing."
—*Dr. Maynard Murray*

SEA-90 sea solids fertilizer has been successfully used for enhancing the growth of wheat fields in Nebraska. Charles Walters, author of *Fertility from the Ocean Deep,* shares the testimony of a Nebraska farmer who found his wheat crop grew in stronger, fuller, and matured earlier....

> **"That wheat was the best wheat I ever grew. It came out of the soil. It covered the hill like hair on a dog's back."**

Regarding sea solids fertilizer for wheat, Walters also mentions...

> **"Used in wheat fields in selenium or molybdenum excess areas, sea solids seem to govern uptake of the excess, making the wheat commercially useable on otherwise condemned acres."**

Sea Solids Fertilization Pioneer Passionate About "Capturing" Ocean for Agriculture

Dr. Murray, M.D., former physician and physiologist, and author of *Sea Energy Agriculture*, was *enthralled* by the nourishing and wellness aspects of the sea and the marvelous unsurpassed health of the marine life. He hoped it was possible that the new field of "transferring this wellness" through sea solids usage for agriculture, could possibly lead to the end of disease and famine.

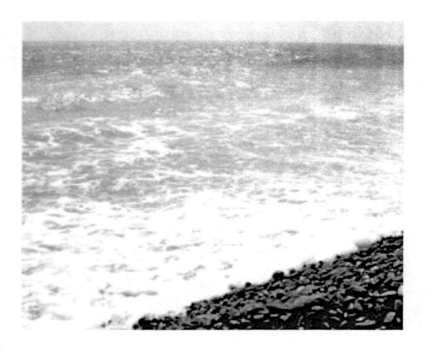

This unique humanitarian believed that all minerals and trace elements found in the effervescent ocean—a bountiful treasure chest, are *all* necessary, *in some way*, to our physiological well-being, our immune systems, and our mental health.

> **"Since the sea foods are, as a group, so valuable a source of the fat-soluble activators, they have been found to be efficient throughout the world not only for controlling tooth decay, but for producing a human stock of high vitality."**
> —*Dr. Weston A. Price*

Dr. Murray envisioned sea energy agriculture being a solution to a looming crisis in agriculture and food production. He said...

"Life is far too short for one person to selfishly guard any new facts he discovers....

"Many minds are better than one, and it is my ardent hope that from this beginning more enthusiasm will be generated which will bring active, probing minds into the field. The results of my beginning research must be amplified and technologically developed in order to best serve mankind."

Perfectly Fed Ocean Life Requires
No Added Fertilizers or Chemicals

Man does not need to fertilize or add chemicals to our oceans to keep the sea life (animals and plants) in better shape, or to protect the sea life from destructive opportunistic microorganisms. The late Dr. Murray found the wondrous ocean life "bathing" in the liquid briny elixir, to be kept *spectacularly* nourished, disease resistant, and healthy.

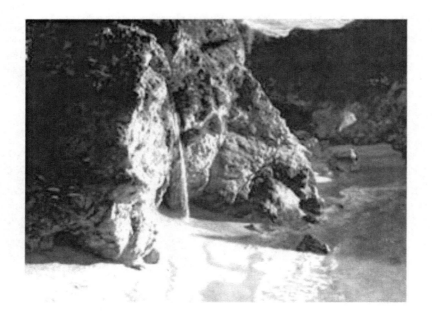

> **"On a worldwide basis then, about 4 billion tons of dissolved material are carried to the sea by rivers each year. The most soluble elements are first picked up by rainwater and that is the reason why sodium chloride (common table salt) is so scarce on land, yet abundant in the sea."**
> —*Dr. Maynard Murray*

We do not need to try to develop disease resistant sea plants because they are *already* largely disease resistant attributed to the perfect and consistent salty chemical arrangement in the natural and pure ocean environment, as Dr. Murray discovered. On the other hand, Dr. Murray said...

> **"The extreme opposite is true on land, where even plants that are grown a few feet apart exhibit chemical differences, especially evident in the micro or trace elements."**

This is why I love to naturally indulge my wheatgrass with this ocean-like solution. I prefer my wheatgrass to be *powerfully* fed, like the potpourri of marine life immersed in the vast expanse of the miraculous sea that take in its flavorful seasoning.

Wheatgrass truly enjoys "devouring" the full splendor of balanced minerals and trace elements that are precisely and healthfully formulated in the life promoting sea.

Aging Process Did Not Seem to Appear in Sea Animals Immersed in Salty Fluid

It was about in 1936 that the late Dr. Murray was tremendously impressed by the high disease resistance of animals in the sea—especially as compared to those on land. At the time, he noted the *shocking* absence of disease in the sea and also the wonderful vitality of the sea animals.

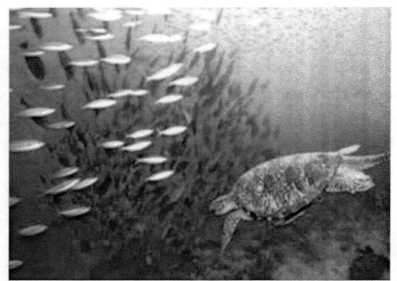

Seawater contains every existing mineral in liquid form.

He theorized that land life had more disease from consuming mineral depleted and weaker plants from mineral deficient soils. Dr. Murray said...

"There is no chronic disease to be found among fish and animal life in the sea that compares to those on land."

This exemplary researcher, who also had a passion for growing plants hydroponically, noted the aging process did not seem to appear or exist with the sea animals he studied.

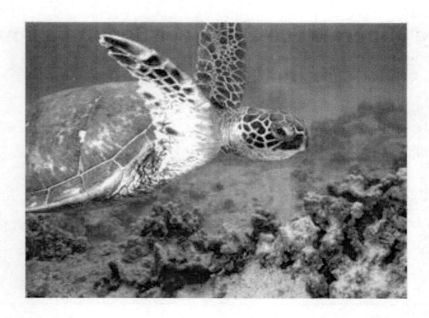

For example, at the time of his research, he was surprisingly unable to find cancer, hardening of the arteries, or arthritis in sea turtles in the pure and untainted ocean—with its smorgasbord of naturally balanced minerals. Dr. Murray imparted...

"It is also known that all land animals develop arteriosclerosis, yet sea animals have never been diagnosed as arteriosclerotic."

Sea Minerals Eco-Fertilizer Benefits Plants, Animals, and Humans

Dr. Murray decided to carefully harvest this seemingly perfect mineral and trace element arrangement circulating in the ocean and then feed it to lucky plants.

He reasoned that if the sea environment could maintain such a high level of disease resistance and be highly supportive of sea *life*, then perhaps its "magical essence" could be fed to plants on land—which could then also greatly benefit. His reasoning was sound....

> **"By properly harvesting sea mineral solids from the ocean, and using those unrefined sea solids as a soil amendment, he found he could *most definitely* bestow the fertility and health promoting legacy of the ocean to plants on land as well."**

Dr. Murray personally experienced *remarkable* success growing plants that were fertilized with sea solids. In fact, as his research continued, he captivatingly found that not only did the sea solids fertilized plants benefit, but the animals fortunate enough to then eat those mineral rich foods, experienced very desirable health improvements as well.

Remineralization Benefits

Plants Benefit with Sea Solids
- Plants flourished
- Increased disease resistance—predators are drawn to weaker, malnourished plants
- Improved crop yields
- Less need for other fertilizers, insecticides, fungicides, herbicides
- Improved taste, sweeter tasting from increased plant sugars
- Faster growth
- Healthier
- Longer shelf life
- Increased protein in alfalfa

Animals Benefit From Eating Plants Fertilized with Sea Solids
- Chickens exhibited perfect health
- Improved reproduction and fertility
- Improved immunity
- Increased disease resistance
- Steers showed weight gain while eating less food (appreciated in farming)
- Animals *delighted* in salted crop fields
- Exhibited more shiny, lush, sleek coats
- More calm, less nervous
- Increased protein, butterfat in livestock

Cancer Bred Mice Doubled their Life Span with Sea Mineral Solids Fertilized Foods

Dr. Murray conducted feeding experiments using sea mineral solids fertilized foods with C3H mice that carried the MMTV, and with rats. (C3H mice are used in research because they always (100%) develop breast cancer, and MMTV stands for mouse mammary tumor virus.)

He made it clear these experiments were conducted on C3H mice and rats, and not humans. Nevertheless, the impressive results indicated a possible way to increase disease resistance and improve health through sea solids fertilized agriculture, and begged for further research. Following, are two of his studies.

In one study, he decided to work with 400 female C3H mice specifically bred to develop breast cancer which would bring about their demise. He broke the C3H mice into two groups—200 mice in each group. One control group was fed regular foods and the other experimental group was fed foods fertilized with sea solids. The control group of mice all died within eight months and seven days (they have a life expectancy of *no more* than nine months).

The experimental mice that were fed foods fertilized with unprocessed sea solids with attached minerals and trace elements, all lived until they were sacrificed at 16 months: **Testing showed no cancerous tissue at that time.**

Life Span Doubled for Cancer Bred C3H Mice Fed Sea Solids Fertilized Foods

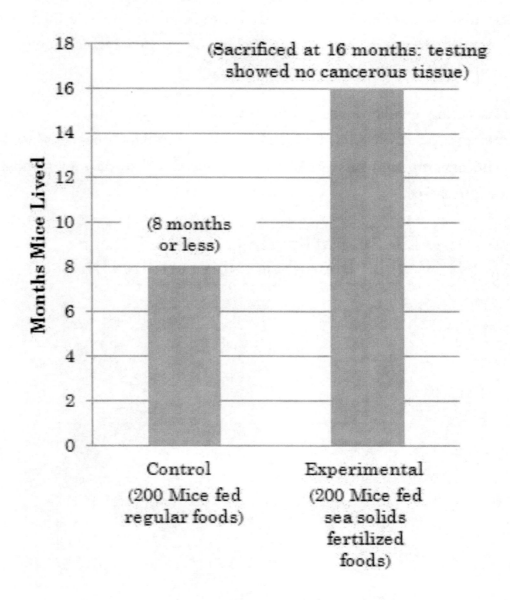

Rats Injected with Cancer Lived Longer with Sea Solids Remineralized Foods

Dr. Murray also experimented with 50 Sprague Dolly rats. All of the rats were injected with cancer (Jensen Carcino-Sarcoma) —shown to be 100% fatal. He then divided the 50 rats into two groups of 25. The control rats were fed regular food, while the experimental rats were fed sea solids fertilized food.

All the rats eating regular foods perished within 21 days. Nine of the rats in the experimental group fed sea solids fertilized foods lived 19 days longer, for 40 days. The remaining 16 experimental rats (64%) were sacrificed at 150 days or 5 months, and found to be cancer free.

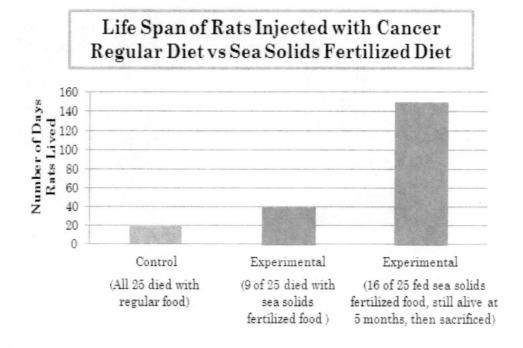

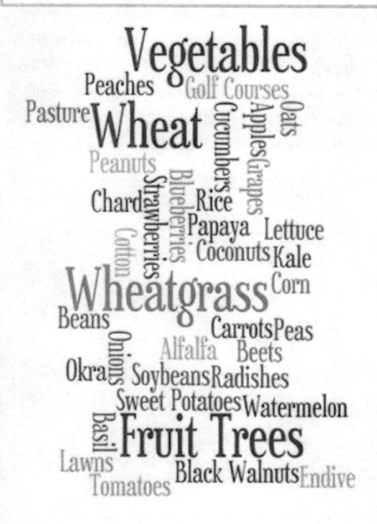

Valuable Ocean Minerals and Trace Elements are Translocated to Sea Solids

In ocean samples taken all over the world, Dr. Murray personally found 90 plus water soluble minerals and trace elements *always* in constant relation and ratio to one another, similar to Johan Forchhammer, even if the salinity (*total amount* of those elements) increased or decreased. He said the trace element ratios in sea water are almost the same as the trace element ratios in blood. After the seawater evaporates, these *liquefied* elements in the ocean *solidify*, and are then found in the sea solids.

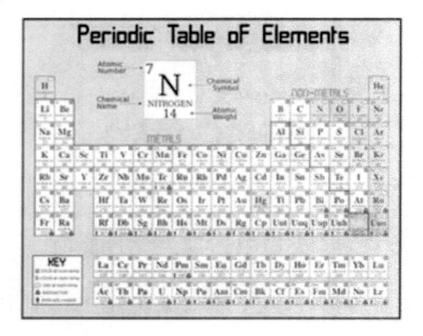

Could it be the *perfect* consistency, balance, and proportion of the full compilation of these periodic table of liquefied elements present in the ocean water are the *ideal* solution for the growth and support of both sea plants *and* land plants (given the right salinity); and subsequently, *tremendously* beneficial to those that eat these foods? I believe so.

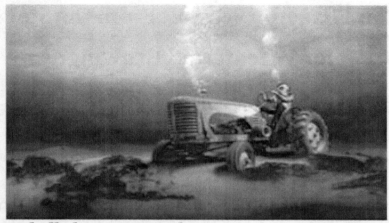

Dr. Murray found all elements on planet Earth are found in the sea solids—with possible exception of some of the gases.

Using mineral rich sea solids as a fertilizer, the wheatgrass can happily uptake this full rainbow of health supporting elements.

> **"Grass is the number one plant in terms of being able to absorb *each and every* mineral and trace element from the soil."**

This makes fertilizing your growing wheatgrass with a sea solids and water solution, and then consuming its juice, so very rewarding and replenishing!

Can I Use Any Sea Salt From the Store for Wheatgrass Growing?

You *can* use unrefined sea salt from the store for wheatgrass growing. But be careful, as even *refined* and element lacking salt can confusingly be labeled as *Sea Salt* at the grocery or health food store, because all salt *originates* from the sea.

You certainly do not want to use refined, element depleted sea salt as a wheatgrass fertilizer. The more naturally proportioned elements in your sea salt fertilizer, the better your harvest. Huge differences exist between different salts as communicated in the salt comparison chart I'll present in a bit.

> **"SEA-90 Sea Solids at SeaAgri.com are listed by the USDA National Organic Program and the Organic Materials Review Institute (OMRI) for use in the production of organic food, fiber, and livestock."**

I experimented with several different salts (marketed as food seasoning), along with SEA-90 sea solids, for wheatgrass growing. I experienced especially good results with SEA-90, which is superior for all the reasons explained in this chapter. It is ideal for wheatgrass growing and gardens.

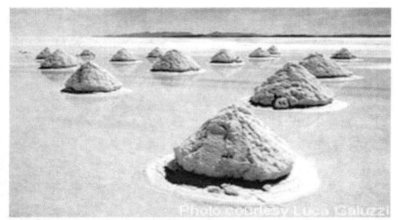

Sea Salt mounds in Bolivia have natural grayish hue.

If you are unable to obtain the SEA-90, look for another sea salt with off-white, grayish or tan coloring (not white), and that originated from evaporated *fresh* ocean water. Learn as much about the company as you can to understand their harvesting methods—you want as many minerals and trace elements as possible to best capture the entire nourishing synergy of the ocean.

You can certainly mix-and-match your fertilizer choices. You can use your fertilizer choices *along with* the sea solids. If you want an outstanding ocean based fertilizer that is affordable, highly valuable, safe, easy to store, simple to apply, and 100% soluble, I absolutely recommend using the SEA-90 sea solids. I will be sharing the recipe for making your sea mineral solids fertilizer in Chapter 7.

SEA-90 Sea Solids Mineral Supplements
In a League of Their Own

Dr. Murray specifically named these salty grains SEA-90 sea solids. They are large crystal grains of salt (basically water soluble rock dust) *and* biological components. All the elements in sea water once came from rock. When the transforming sea solids are combined with water and liquefied, the elements are then immediately available for plant uptake. Hopefully they won't mistakenly become confused with the huge variety of different sea salts on the market with their differing amounts of minerals and trace elements.

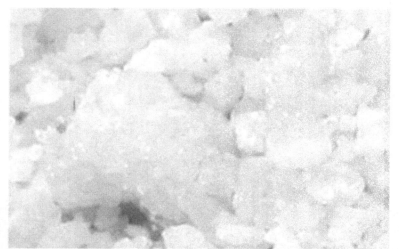

Off-white crystal grains have their own unique shape and size.

The 90+ minerals and trace elements in sea solids are *perfectly balanced* by Mother Nature herself. The mineral and trace element balance, ratios, and content of SEA-90 mineral solids are essentially the same as the sea water from which they were created. **No minerals or trace elements have been removed, leached, or weathered away from them.**

According to Dr. Murray, there is no sea salt available anywhere that compares to the SEA-90 sea mineral solids harvested at the special and pristine location he discovered. He searched the planet and found only three perfect locations where he knew he could obtain and diligently harvest sea solids to preserve their buffet of minerals and trace elements—the foundation for life.

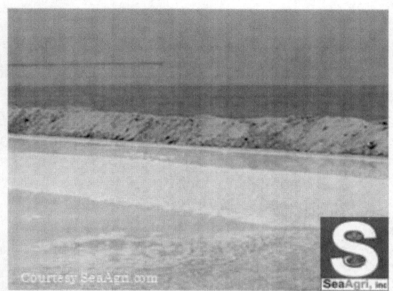

SEA-90 sea solids are drying in foreground and are formed during solar evaporation. Dissolved salts (elements) crystallize out of the liquid ocean.

If you use other sea salt besides the SEA-90 sea solids for wheatgrass growing, you will not be getting the entire mineral and trace elements *and* biological package, and your results will vary.

SEA-90 sea solids are available at SeaAgri.com.

All Salt Originates From the Sea

A Salty Comparison Chart

	Refined Salt
Ingredients	Sodium Chloride plus additives which can include: anti-caking agents, bleaching agents, aluminum derivates, sugar, fluoride, potassium iodide. (Additives do not need to be on label.) 93% used for industrial purposes, remaining used in food business, especially preservative in processed foods
Color and shape	White; small grain for easy pouring
Located	Salt mines on land or ocean
Processing method	Varies
Element status	Elements are stripped and sold to industry
Notes	Can be referred to as white poison; inflammatory, unnatural, unwholesome food

	Unrefined Salt
Ingredients	Sodium chloride along with accompanied elements, read label for any additives

* I select unrefined sea salts for seasoning my foods, preferring gray, sun dehydrated sea salt from fresh ocean water to best retain minerals and elements in balanced proportion as found in ocean, with no additives, tested for pollutants. |
Color and shape	Usually white, pinkish, or gray. Black or red sea salts can get their color from added activated charcoal, or red clay; grain size varies
Located	Salt mines on land or ocean
Processing method	Varies
Element status	Some elements can be missing depending on processing method and where obtained, or could have been rinsed or weathered away
Notes	Can be referred to as white gold; anti-inflammatory, healing, natural, nourishing

	SEA-90 Sea Solids
Ingredients	Sodium chloride along with accompanied 90+ balanced minerals and trace elements–no additives, tested for pollutants * Ideal for wheatgrass growing and gardening (when combined with water, the elements become isotonic and *immediately* available for plant to absorb)
Color and shape	Tan or gray – Off-white color indicates retaining of darker trace elements; grain size varies
Located	Ocean
Processing method	Sun dehydrated and harvested from fresh seawater
Element status	Care is taken to best capture *all* balanced elements in ocean, sea solids protected from rains rinsing away valuable elements
Notes	Harvested from sea to capture complete spectrum of minerals and trace elements for fertilization

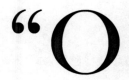"On average, grasses produce three or four times more roots by weight than they do leaves and stems, giving them a root-to-shoot ratio that is ten times as high as that of a forest."

—Candace Savage
Prairie: A Natural History

Chapter 6: Growing Wheatgrass Instructions (Method One)

"Every disease is a sign of a lack of certain chemical elements. No disease can exist unless there is a lack of chemical elements in the body."

—Bernard Jensen
The Healing Power of Chlorophyll from Plant Life

Rinse Seeds Before Soaking Them

I will now give instructions on how to grow one tray (21" x 11" x 2") of wheatgrass. You understand the wheatgrass growing tools needed, the importance of good soil and compost, the high value of sea solids fertilizer, and why good wheat seed selection matters. So let's continue...

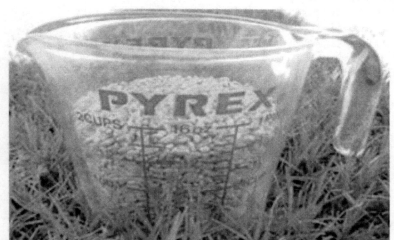

Use 1 ½ cups or 12 ounces of seeds per growing tray.

The unseen microbial world is quite fascinating. As said, there are actually microscopic critters like fungi and bacteria on the surface of those cute little wheat seeds. Therefore, pre-rinsing and pre-soaking the seeds is of value. Healthier seeds harbor almost no fungi.

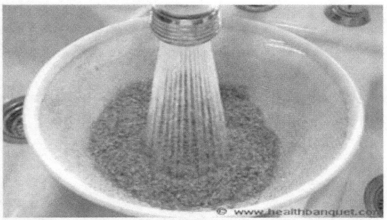

It is best not to allow the seeds down the drain so they don't start sprouting in your pipes.

117

First, start by rinsing 1 1/2 cups (about 12 ounces) of seed *before* soaking:

• Move seeds around while rinsing—a **thirty second** rinse in lukewarm water is fine

• Will reduce non-beneficial fungi and bacteria on surface of seed that can lead to increased mold

• Will notice less mold by including important pre-rinsing step

• Adjust the amount of seeds based on your wheatgrass tray size—increasing the amount of seeds will create more dense growth

Rinse Seeds, Soak Seeds, Rinse Seeds

When rinsing wheat seeds, they will lodge in strainers with larger holes.

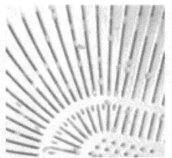

**Seeds easily lodge in a strainer with wider slots or holes,
thus making cleanup time longer.**

So make sure to use a sieve or strainer with smaller openings, or line the strainer with a cheesecloth. The cleanup will be easier and the grains will be more quickly transferred.

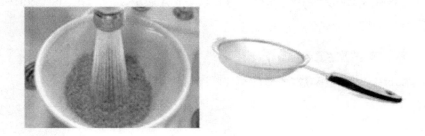

Next, transfer those pre-rinsed seeds into a bowl. Put roughly three times as much water as you have seeds into the bowl. Plus, add to water the recommended whole sea solids along with the soaking seeds. (You *can* use another unrefined sea salt in this soaking step. For the main fertilizing though, you will receive the best results with SEA-90 sea solids.) The nutritious sea solids will strengthen the soaking seeds, help decrease mold, increase germination of seeds, and increase vigor of the sprouts:

• Add 4 1/2 cups water and 1 1/2 cups seeds to soaking bowl

• Add enough water for seeds to absorb and to stay immersed—seeds will expand to twice their size

• **Add 1 teaspoon whole sea solids into bowl of 4 1/2 cups water and 1 1/2 cups seeds, stir to dissolve**

• Increase or decrease sea solids if using more seeds with more water or less seeds with less water

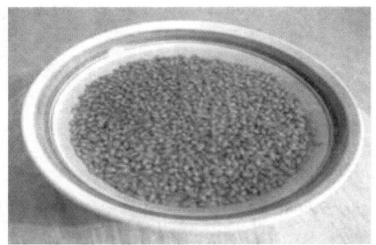

Seeds are soaking in water and sea solids.

Soaking supports germination. Overnight or day soak is fine:

• 6 - 8 hours in the warmer summer when the benefits of soaking occur at a more rapid pace

• 8 - 12 hours in the winter

• After soaking, rinse seeds *again*, 15 - 30 second rinse is fine

Plant Seeds in Tray With Good Drainage

These plastic trays are perfect for planting your pre-soaked wheat seeds. You can certainly select your own different preferred growing trays. I am showing you the growing trays and tray set up I have found to work successfully.

Wheatgrass grows best in a tray or growing container with good drainage. Therefore, if you are using these shown black plastic growing trays, make sure you place your soil and plant your seeds in the tray *with* drainage slots. Note the white arrows pointing to a few tray drainage slots in the photo.

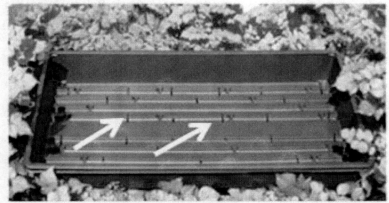

Tray with slots and dimensions of 21" x 11" x 2" works well.

I recommend purchasing 1 - 2 sets of wheatgrass trays *with* slots *and* 1 - 2 sets of wheatgrass trays *without* slots, depending on how many wheatgrass trays you will be growing at one time. Each set comes with 5 trays. If needed, I have a growing wheatgrass supplies store at HealthBanquet.com. You may also be able to find them at a local nursery.

> **"Each tray produces about 12 - 15 ounces of wheatgrass juice. The amount of juice can vary with density, moisture, length of grass, and extraction ability of juicer."**

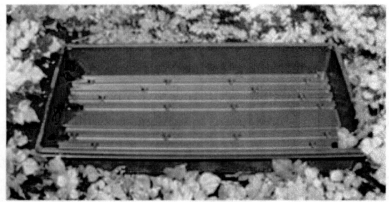

Here is tray without slots and dimensions of 21" x 11" x 2".

You *can* plant in a tray with *no* slots or holes, but wheatgrass grows best with good drainage provided by having slots in the bottom of your selected growing tray. Growing trays work nicely because they are shallow and can hold the perfect amount of soil to grow a beautiful batch of wheatgrass.

Place Tray with Drainage Inside Non-Drainage Tray

Next, double up trays by placing wheatgrass growing tray *with* slots directly *inside* of wheatgrass tray with *no* slots.

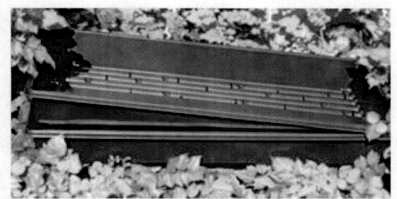

Top tray with slots fits perfectly in bottom tray with no slots.

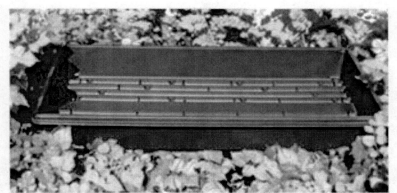

Tray w*ith* slots is resting inside tray *without* slots.

This doubling up of trays will lengthen the lifespan of the plastic trays. You don't have to double up your trays. I did not at first, but you will appreciate less mess on your kitchen counter through doubling up with the *no slot* tray on the bottom. If you decide *not* to double up your trays, but want to plant your wheat seeds in a single tray *with* drainage slots, you can line the bottom of tray with one layer of paper towels for less mess on your counter, though there can *still* be drainage onto your counter.

Make sure to dump out excess water that over accumulates in that bottom *no slot* tray during the watering process. If you feel the top tray is not draining into the bottom tray as well as you would like, feel free to place some kind of spacer between the top and bottom tray. It is not necessary, but it will assist drainage.

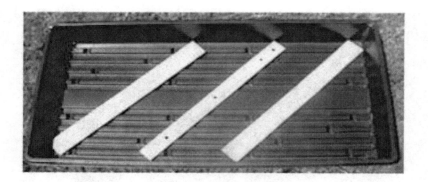

I have used a couple flat pieces of wood as a spacer before—similar to the dimensions of a ruler. A spacer roughly 1/4 inches thick is fine. This gives the top tray a little lift up and off the bottom tray, thus allowing the water to more freely drain.

You Can Pre-Fill Trays with Soil

To continue, place your soil in the growing tray. You can spread from 1" to 1 1/2" of good soil in your growing tray. I usually lean toward 1" of soil, as I believe that amount is sufficient to grow excellent wheatgrass. I like to grow my wheatgrass in soil, Mother Earth herself, just as Ann Wigmore preferred. Spread out the soil smoothly. You want a nice flat surface for placing your wheatgrass seeds.

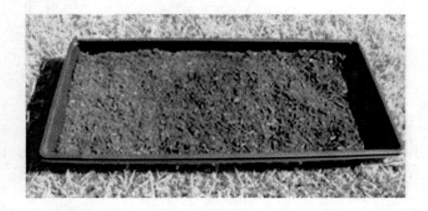

Here is a tip to save time. Once you have your soil available, you may want to pre-fill some growing trays. In other words, put the soil in several growing trays at one time. If you make a few of these growing trays up ahead of time, this will save you time and clean-up from individually preparing them each time you want to grow a tray of wheatgrass.

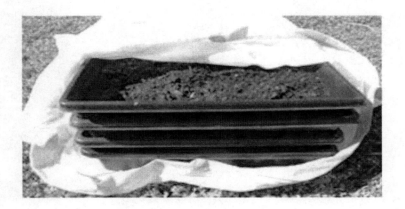

If you decide to pre-fill several trays beforehand, simply place the soil in your trays, the tray *with* the slots. Then stack the trays individually inside a large plastic garbage bag that you can close off from the air—to keep the soil from drying out.

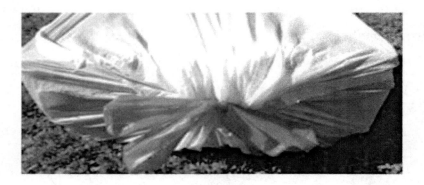

When you are ready to plant, open up the bag, take out your tray with soil, place it inside a second tray with *no slots,* and place it on your counter or area of your choice, and proceed with growing instructions. You can *initially* double up your trays and then stack and store them in the bag. However, just remember to wipe off that bottom tray that has been sitting in soil, before you place it on your counter. Or, skip the bag entirely, but soil may dry out and need extra water before planting seeds.

Place Pre-Soaked Seeds on Soil

Alright, take your pre-rinsed, pre-soaked, and post-rinsed seeds and place them on top of the soil.

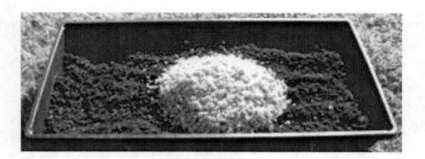

Just smooth out the seeds evenly all over your bed of soil, including corners and edges:
- Seeds will touch each other but will not be piled on top of other seeds
- No harm is done if they are so close to each other that they slightly overlap; you will get a more dense growth
- When spreading seeds on soil, I like to have them get into contact and rub around in the wonderful *protective* soil to lightly coat the surface of the seed—actually mix seeds amongst the soil a bit, keeping the seeds on the surface of the soil
- Try to spread seeds so there is a nice *flat* surface of them, so they will be more evenly watered
- You can lightly pat them into place in the soil

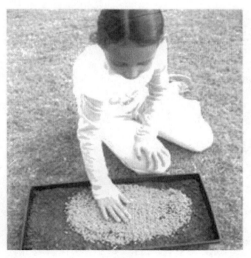

Again, if you have chosen to use more seeds per tray, say the 2 cups of seeds versus the 1 1/2 cups of seeds, then it will be more densely covered with growing blades of wheatgrass:

• With use of 1 1/2 cups of seed per tray, wheatgrass growth is less dense, thus more air circulation and less mold

• With 2 cups of seeds per tray there is higher density, but increased risk of mold

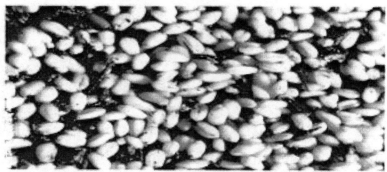

Seeds spread out evenly on top of soil.

Amount of Required Watering May Vary

This is how it will look when your seeds are dispersed evenly, in preparation for watering.

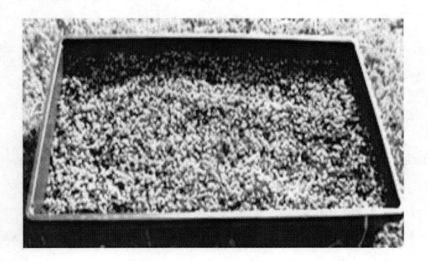

When it comes to watering, there is room for adaptation on your part. The amount and intervals of watering for wheatgrass growing are not "set in stone." Needed watering depends on many factors:

- Amount, moisture level, and depth of soil in growing tray
- Season, temperature, and humidity in growing area
- Type of growing tray used—size, good drainage or not

For basic watering, you can use the watering vessel of your choice. It is not the watering container that is important; it is the *actually applied* amount of water that matters. To hydrate my wheatgrass during its lifespan, I use different approaches: a pump water sprayer, watering can, measuring cup, occasionally the kitchen faucet, or maybe even the outdoor hose with a spray nozzle if my wheatgrass happens to be outside.

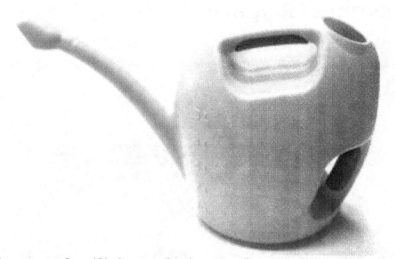

**Pre-make your fertilizing solution and store it in a watering can
or pump sprayer for future use.**

As mentioned, I am a big fan of using the sea solids and water for not only soaking my seeds, but for fertilizing the growing wheatgrass as well. Almost always during the soaking, sprouting, and final wheatgrass growing stage (the entire growing process), when using water, I add sea solids to the water because of its many benefits.

Soaking seeds and fertilizing with sea solids and water is a highly valuable choice, but it is not necessary.

First Watering is About 2 Cups of Water
Per Growing Tray

After the pre-soaked seeds are atop your soil, they and the soil beneath them are ready to be moistened.

In this first watering, **give them *about* 2 cups sea solids and water solution per growing tray** (enough to moisten seeds and soil directly below seeds). This solution is easily applied with a watering can or sprayer. Again, I share this excellent fertilizing solution recipe in Chapter 7.

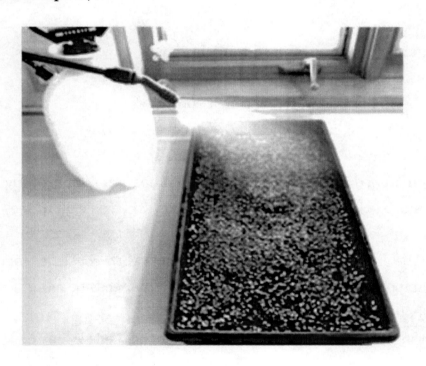

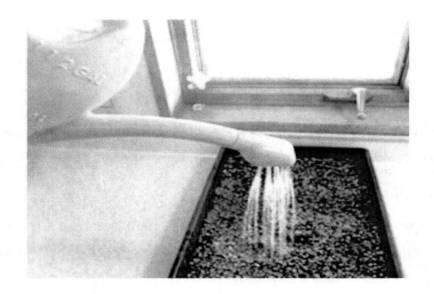

This initial watering can be any time during the day:

- Tap water is OK, filtered water is better

- Water can be applied via watering can or sprayer

- If using watering can, move quickly to avoid over watering

- Seeds need to stay moistened during sprouting stage

- Moisten soil *immediately* below seeds too, in preparation for growing roots

- The more moist soil, right underneath the seeds, will also help to keep the seedlings from drying out

- Soil should be nicely moistened, a bit damp—not overly soaked or muddy

- It is more important that the soil *directly under* the seeds be more moist, than the soil toward bottom of tray

- After watering, it may be necessary to rearrange the seeds evenly on top of the soil again

Place Plastic Cover on Seeds

After this initial watering, place a cover tray *with slots* directly on top of the bottom tray of seeds as shown in the picture.

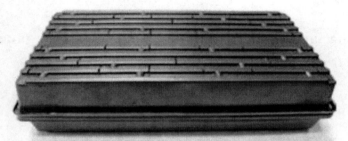

Cover with slots sets atop bottom tray with seeds.

If you place a cover on top *without slots*, place that cover slightly off to the side (1/2 - 3/4 inches) so as to allow in a little air.

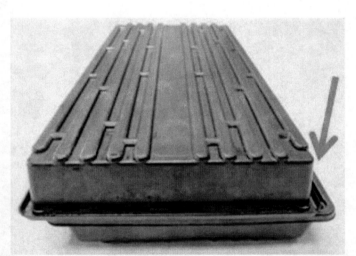

**If using a cover without slots, place it slightly ajar
so more air can reach the seeds.**

These covers provide a nice germinating environment:

    • Help to simulate outdoor growing conditions—seeds kept more moist, comfortably warm, and protected from light as they would be if outdoors under a light layer of soil

    • Both cover with slots *and* cover without slots placed slightly ajar and above bottom tray, will each allow in a bit of air, thus helping with mold reduction

During these first few days of sprouting in this incubative environment, you want to keep the seeds *moistened* for increased germination. However, it is very important not to over water them during this sprouting stage.

If the seeds experience more stressful sprouting conditions from too much water or they dry out from not enough water, their growth will be negatively impacted.

Both over watering and *under* watering can negatively impact your sprouting wheatgrass.

Pump Sprayer Better Controls Applied Amount of Water

About 24 hours after the initial watering, remove the cover temporarily and <u>mist</u> all the seeds. Then replace cover. **You want the seeds kept moist, but not soggy.**

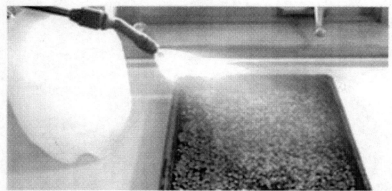

FloMaster sprayer holds water and sea solids fertilizer.

I use the pump sprayer to mist the seeds during the more sensitive sprouting stage, and up until the wheatgrass is about one inch tall. From that point of growth forward, when the blades of grass are about one inch tall, they desire more water. You can also slightly turn the end tip of the black spray nozzle to shoot out a narrow *stream* of water, or you can use a watering can. It is faster to apply more water with the watering can.

You may find you just want to use a pump sprayer, or maybe just a watering can throughout the hydrating process. You can certainly mix and match according to your preferences.

This easy-to-operate one gallon pump pressure sprayer provides a nice gentle mist for your sprouting seeds. You certainly *can* use a smaller *manual* hand spray bottle, if it works best for your wheatgrass growing situation and storage space.

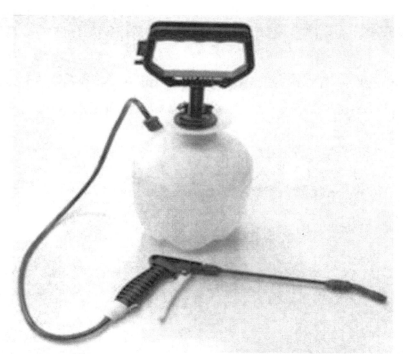

Pre-make your fertilizing solution and store in sprayer for future use.

However, the pump pressure sprayer is far easier—no more continuous pulling of the handle on the manual spray bottles. Especially if you have several trays of wheatgrass growing at one time, you will appreciate a pump sprayer. Several pumps will provide a lengthy spraying of the mist.

Watering is Like a Gentle Cleansing Rain

Please use your better judgment in determining how much and when to mist your sprouting seeds. Your growing climate and personal experience will help you determine the right amount of misting for your new and more vulnerable forming sprouts. Here in the Southwest, I usually lightly mist all the growing sprouts 1 - 2 times per day.

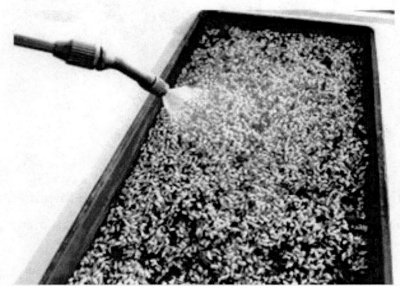

You want the sprouting seeds kept moist, but not soggy.

To continue, if your seedlings need misting, lightly mist all of them with the water and sea solids solution. You can use plain water, but you will have better results with the sea solids and water fertilizer. Misting the seeds during their sprouting stage will also help keep the mold down from its cleansing abilities.

The seeds are more sensitive during the first few days of their sprouting stage, so you will need to be more fastidious with your watering care. Using a spray bottle or pump sprayer for misting them, will give you better watering control. Only a light misting to keep them moistened is necessary during the first few days of the sprouting stage, as their root system is not yet established.

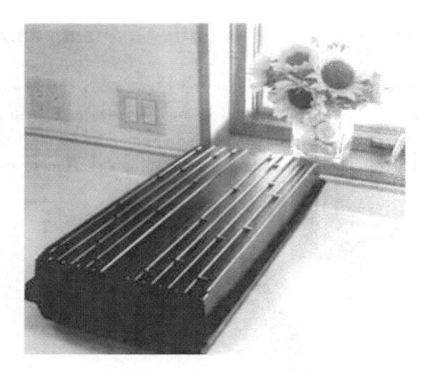

Each day when the seeds are sprouting and up until they are forming into grass that is about one inch high, you can mist them 1 - 2 times per day. After misting, put the cover back on.

Permanently Remove Cover After Sprouting Stage

In a few days, when the great majority of those seeds have put forth pale yellow sprouts that are turning into blades of grass and that are about one inch in height, **remove the cover permanently**. Keep in mind, some seeds may never germinate. The new wheatgrass is now ready to be exposed to the indirect sunlight.

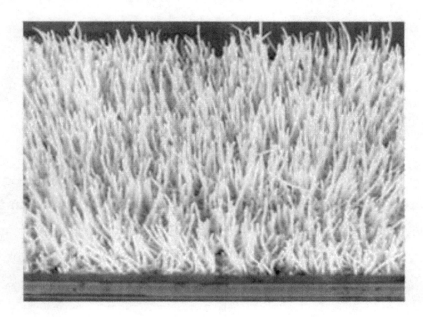

There may be a few latent seeds that have not sprouted out yet, or are just beginning to sprout. Still go ahead and remove the lid at this time. Keeping the cover on top of the sprouting seeds for longer than a few days, decreases the oxygen level to them for a longer time, and can contribute to more mold.

You may get busy sometimes, and not get around to taking off the lid when the baby grass is about one inch tall. It is fine if you don't take the lid off at the *exact* perfect time. Just proceed forward with your wheatgrass growing steps. But do be aware, with the cover in place for too long, the chance of mold increases.

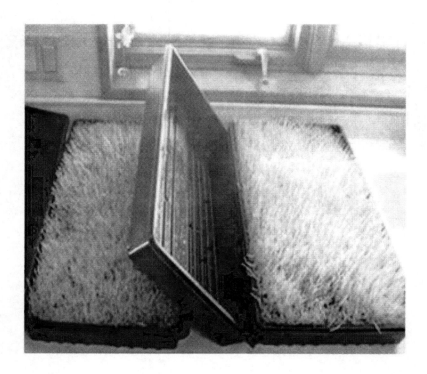

When the covered growing wheatgrass has not received any (or minimal) sunlight, it will appear pale yellow in color. After permanently removing the cover, and after a few days of sunlight, it will gradually turn into a beautiful emerald green color.

Root System Strongly Supports Wheatgrass

Once the seeds are done sprouting and they have officially started turning into baby blades of grass (about one inch high), their root system is becoming established and they are not so vulnerable to growing imperfections.

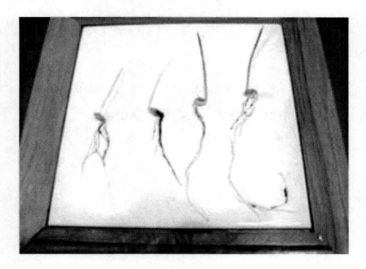

The wheatgrass develops an elaborate labyrinth of roots, seeking out every possible nook and cranny to voraciously consume the water and nutrients. The extensive ever-working root system also helps to keep the wheatgrass more resilient.

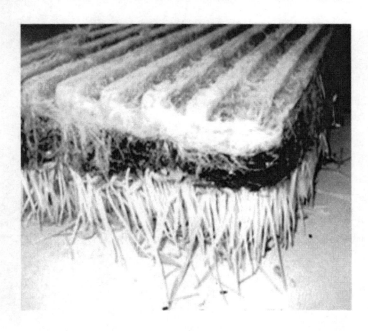

If the wheatgrass does not receive water at the perfect time, it now has a massive intertwining jungle of roots that seek out already existing water to help hold it over. The wheat *grass* is far less sensitive than the sprouting seed, and if it is *over* watered, good drainage should help solve an excess application.

In other words, you no longer have to be as conscientious about providing the right amount of water when the wheatgrass is a couple of inches tall, and the root system is distributed well throughout the tray.

Also now, it is much easier for the wheatgrass to be able to withstand temperatures outside of its ideal growing range of **65° - 75°** Fahrenheit.

Watering Can Quickly Applies Water When Grass is 1 – 2 Inches Tall or Higher

Now that the sprouting stage is basically complete and the uncovered growing grass is taller, one inch or higher, and more dense, you can use a watering can with the sea solids fertilizer solution to water it—each time from now up until harvest.

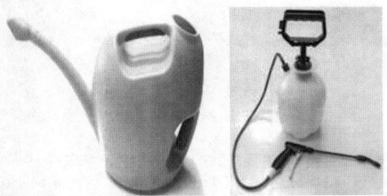

If space, you can store watering containers on towel inside nearby cabinet.

Since the longer blades of wheatgrass and their increasing root system like more water now, hydrating will be more quickly accomplished with a watering can than with the sprayer.

If you choose, of course it is fine to substitute the sea solids watering solution with just *plain* water, now and then, up until harvest. Personally, once the wheatgrass is about one inch tall, I will occasionally water with just *plain* water. However, my primary source of watering is with the sea solids and water solution.

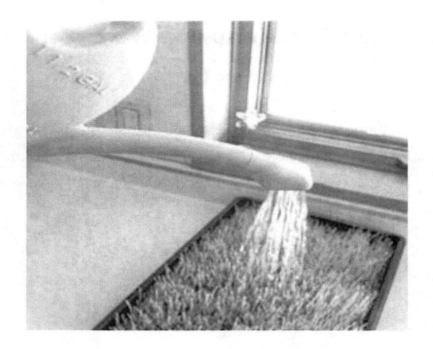

Again, the excellent sea solids and water fertilizer is a simple and affordable way to increase the highly valuable minerals and trace elements in your wheatgrass, and to thus put forth an overall even healthier wheatgrass plant.

"After the sprouting is completed and grass is about one inch tall, continue to water every day, or every other day, until you have harvested your entire batch of wheatgrass. Wheatgrass will appear more moist and succulent, not dried out, if amply watered."

Water Every Day or Every Other Day Until Harvest

In determining watering amount each day henceforth, you will need to take some variables into consideration:

- Amount of sunlight the wheatgrass is getting
- How quickly the wheatgrass is growing
- Temperature and humidity level indoors
- Current moisture level of soil

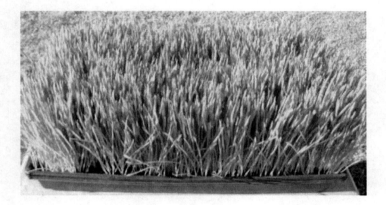

> **"Water enough so the soil is nice and moist, but not muddy. You can water the wheatgrass at any time—day or night."**

As mentioned, your wheatgrass is much more forgiving of watering imperfections, once it has finished the sprouting stage. However, do your best to properly hydrate it during this final growing stage.

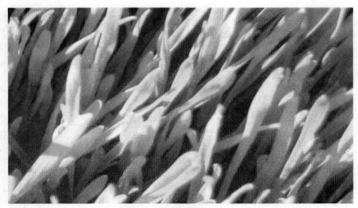

With proper watering, your wheatgrass will reward you with gratitude demonstrated by its more open blades, vitality, cheerful green hue, lusciousness, and beauty—versus having more mold or blades wilting and curling up from dehydration.

Simply, keep the soil nice and moist up until harvest.

Harvest is Ready When 7 - 10 Inches Tall

Begin harvesting your young blades of wheatgrass or barley grass when it is between 7 - 10 inches tall. Wheatgrass is at its *peak* state of nutrition when it is between 7 - 10 inches tall. At this stage, it houses the most enzyme activity, vitamins, chlorophyll, and proteins.

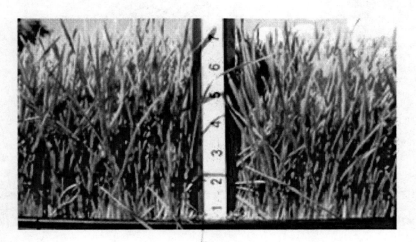

Ann Wigmore also recommended harvesting the wheatgrass when it is between 7 - 10 inches in height:

- **Grass will usually reach this height in about 10 - 14 days**, depending on temperature
- In hot weather, it might reach 10 inches in 5 days

You *can* harvest and consume the juice from your wheatgrass when out of its *peak nutritional* range and still enjoy this green vegetable. Though for optimum nutrients, strive to harvest it between 7 - 10 inches tall.

Once the wheatgrass grows longer than about the 10 inches mark, it starts falling over, yellows, and loses it look of desirability and vibrancy. Also, it doesn't taste as "lively." Strive to consume it in its optimum stage of stored nutritional value and liveliness, when it is emerald green in color and energetically reaching upwards.

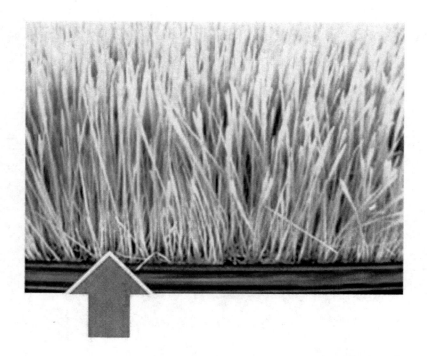

Cut the wheatgrass toward its base, right above the soil line with scissors or a knife. Only cut the amount you plan to juice. Finally, rinse off the wheatgrass, juice, and drink. I demonstrate in a video how to juice wheatgrass with the Hurricane Manual Juicer at HealthBanquet.com. Cheers!

Can I Harvest the Second Growth?

Grass will usually regrow after the first harvest, especially if you have real good soil, but not quite as tall as the first batch. However, I just consume the first growth, as that is when the nutrition is at its peak. You can start a brand new batch after harvesting is complete, or anytime during the growing cycle.

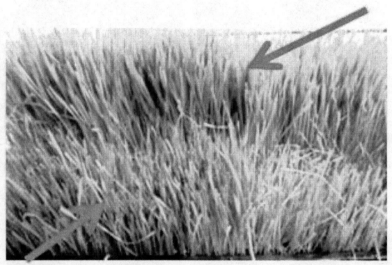

The wheatgrass is growing back in again (second growth) in the front row—after its first harvest. There is an unharvested first growth in the back row.

A healthy regrowth after that first harvest indicates very good soil quality. You can certainly consume the grass from the second or even third regrowth, as it is still providing nutrition. It is just not as high in nutrition and vigor as the first growth, and it tastes slightly bitter—less desirable. The first growth tastes the freshest and sweetest, and appears the most vibrant. Juicing this first growth captures that extra initial nutrition and energy. After harvesting is complete, toss out the consumed mat of wheatgrass (or place in compost bin), clean plastic tray, and replant.

Side note: I have harvested my wheatgrass many times at the six inch mark when I really wanted to consume it, even though it was not at its optimum height. I have even harvested it when 3 - 5 inches tall. Keep in mind, you won't receive as much juice from 4 - 5 inch long wheatgrass, as from 7 - 10 inch long wheatgrass.

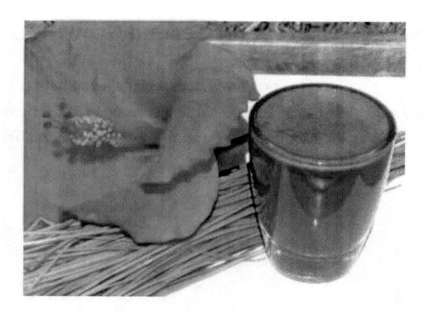

So yes it is optimal between the 7 – 10 inch mark, and from the first harvest. But you can certainly choose to consume it before or after its peak nutritional height.

Grass Growing Stages Pictorial Review

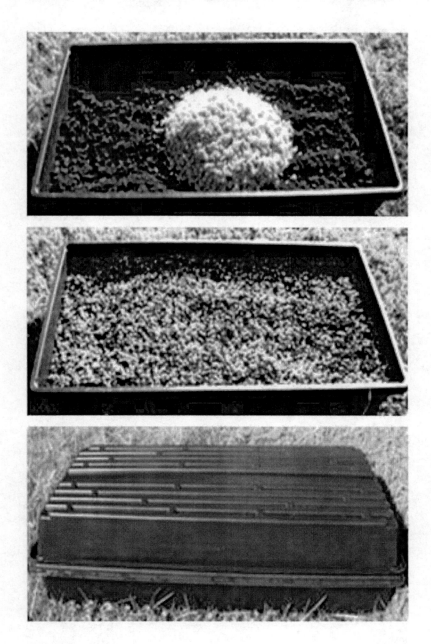

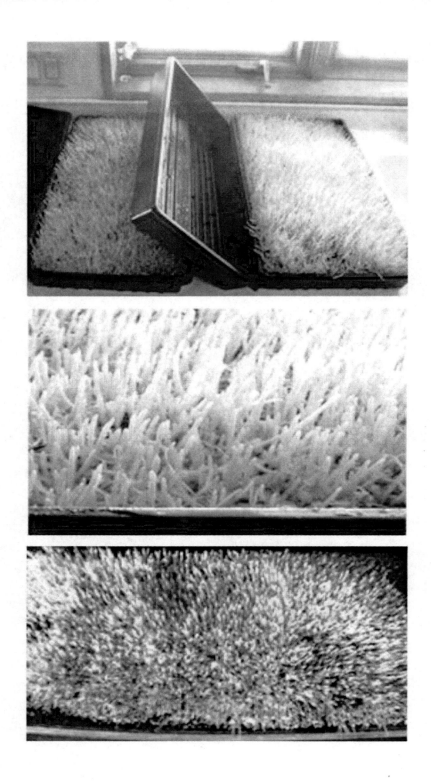

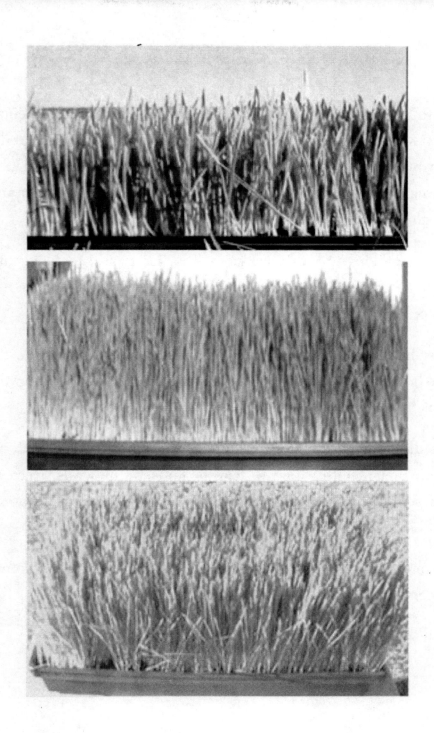

153

Wheatgrass Juice Accompaniments

It is believed to be "ideal" to drink wheatgrass juice straight, without being diluted with other juices or water. However, some simply cannot drink it straight and may become more creative by adding other juices while working toward that "ideal." A benefit to drinking it straight is you are able to more *quickly* drink or sip the tinier amount, than if you had a full glass with other added juices.

When people are looking to regain wellness, it is also typical to avoid eating foods for *about* an hour before and an hour after drinking this juice. Health centers serving wheatgrass juice are more regimented in this way.

Many are just happy and grateful to consume this highly nutritious beverage even though maybe how they choose to mix and match it with other juices, and/or when they choose to drink it, may not be "ideal."

Everyone has different reasons for consuming wheatgrass. Some wish to improve or better maintain their health, some to take in fantastic minerals, trace elements and vitamins, and some because they feel and function better—having more appreciated energy.

If you need some ideas to help counter its flavor, and make its consumption a little easier, the Accompaniments or Chasers Chart will help.

Accompaniments or Chasers

- Carrot juice
- Celery juice
- Pineapple juice
- Grapefruit juice
- Orange juice
- Apple juice
- Your favorite juices
- Coconut water (delicious and easy to add)
- A squeeze of lemon, lemon wedge, juiced sprig of parsley, mint leaves, or basil

Obtain organic if possible to better avoid pesticides that can remain on outside *and* inside of fruit or vegetable.

> **"Today's modern theory that one should eat 'low-fat foods' is incomplete, as these studies were based on inferior and nutritionally worthless fats....**
>
> **"Fats are the substances that govern all life phenomena, which responsibly participate for orderly vital function, growth and absorption of the sun. Vitamins, trace elements etc. offer no aid to a person if he has been harmed by consuming the wrong fats."**
>
> —*Dr. Johanna Budwig*

Side Note: Make sure you are best avoiding bad fats and incorporating the nutrient dense and traditionally consumed good oils and fats into your diet, as they play an *essential* role for good health and help with nutrient absorption. My favorites that I *primarily* consume are non-refined, virgin coconut oil, *real* butter (prefer organic), bottled Carlson Cod Liver Oil, Extra Virgin Olive Oil, and bottled Barlean's Organic Flax Seed Oil.

"We find that a leaf is a very efficient organ of absorption. We find that the materials move into the upper surface of the leaf as well as the lower surface. We find that it enters at night and during the daytime. If we apply it (leaf fertilizing), we find it moves downward through the plant— at the rate of a foot an hour.

"If we apply some of this material to the leaf of a bean plant, the material moves very quickly into all parts of the plant."

—Dr. H. B. Tukey
Head Dept. of Horticulture,
Michigan State College

Chapter 7: Optional Foliar Feeding - How and When to Apply Fertilizer

"Not only can plants absorb nutrients through the roots, but also through the foliage, the fruit, the twigs, the trunk, and even the flowers."

—Dr. H. B. Tukey
Head Dept. of Horticulture,
Michigan State College

Optional Foliar Feeding is a Perfect Fertilization Added Touch

Foliar (of or relating to leaves) feeding is a method of spraying liquid nutrients directly onto the surface area of plant leaves. Foliar feeding is perfectly suited for applying the **100% soluble**, highly absorbable, sea solids and water solution to the leaves of your growing wheatgrass.

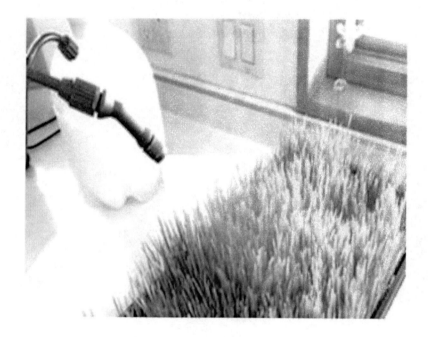

Foliar sprays can increase the nutrient uptake by plants. It is a fantastic and *eminently effective* way for the wheatgrass to take in and translocate those additional natural and perfectly balanced minerals and trace elements from the sea. These valuable dissolved minerals and trace elements pass from the surface of the leaves and then throughout the plant structure to marvelously fortify it.

> **"With foliar applications, nutrients are absorbed rapidly, usually within 6 - 24 hours. The grass leaves can soak up nutrients even faster than roots."**

Foliar spraying with the sea solids solution is an *adjunct* treatment to your sea solids *root* fertilization program. This foliar fertilization opportunity is *optional*.

> **"Material applied to the leaf of a plant can actually quickly travel and concentrate in the growing tips of the roots, which are deep into the soil. Usually these materials gather predominantly in the active growing areas of the plant."**

Foliar feeding is *not* meant to replace a steady soil and root fertilization plan—it **should *enhance* it if you choose to incorporate it.** Certain minerals are better absorbed all *throughout* the plant via the *roots* in the soil. Foliar feeding is more of an insurance policy for *optimal* nutrient uptake and plant growing success.

Foliar Feeding is Easy

Foliar feeding helps to *prevent* growing problems, rather than fix them after they have occurred. Wheatgrass that is in good shape nutritionally will more likely be able to respond to foliar feeding. Foliar spraying with the sea solids solution will:

- Make good wheatgrass even better
- Increase nutrient uptake, correct deficiencies
- Help increase resistance to mold
- Increase its tolerance to stressors like heat and cold
- Strengthen and fortify plant
- Support successful growth

You can *unknowingly* foliar feed your wheatgrass if you water it using the sprayer and sea solids solution. However, I will share clear instructions on how to foliar feed your wheatgrass so you learn the *official* technique and can proceed *knowingly*. Basically, it entails simply *spraying* the sea solids and water fertilizer directly onto your growing leaves of wheatgrass.

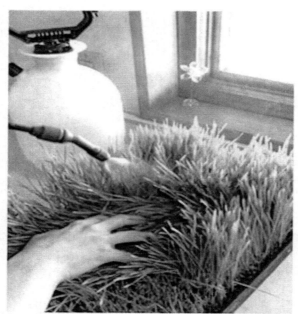

The fertilizer will reach more surface area on the front and back of the wheatgrass blades if you comb through them with your fingers while spraying.

I will elaborate more on this beneficial topic. You can separate the wheatgrass blades with your fingers as you apply the fertilizer to both their front and back surface area. Finely mist them—no need to overly saturate with the liquid fertilizer as too much will more easily drip off the grass leaf blades. It takes only a few seconds to spray all the green blades, and it is a rather enjoyable activity.

> **"Grass and forage is the best medicine."**
> —*Charles Walters*

Wheatgrass Can Absorb Nutrients
From Front and Back of Leaves

The nutrients are absorbed and taken in through the leaves via the permeable epidermis (outer skin surface on leaves) and stomata (plural for stoma). **Stomata are found on both the front and back surface of the leaves (blades) of wheatgrass**. They are tiny multi-purpose, liquid drinking, and "breathing" mouth-like valves. They also kind of look like the pores on your body—except for being green.

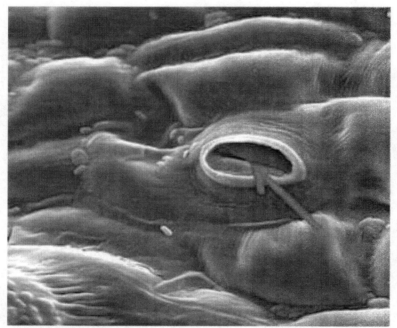

This is a magnified picture of an open stoma on a plant.

There are thousands of stomata found on both the front and back surface of wheatgrass leaves—just slightly less on the backside. In fact, there are about 7,000 stomata per square centimeter on the upper surface of wheatgrass leaves. And barley leaves can have increased stomata density.

When the stomata are open, they let air in and out, and release closely monitored water evaporation. During hot weather, they "perspire" through the stomata to cool down.

These openings take in nutrients that can come from the air, rain, sprinklers, watering cans, and even *more* easily from *fine mist* sprayers.

> "Everybody, the doctor, the sick person who wants to be healthy, we are all part of nature. We must respect this fact. And it is the greatest physicists and quantum biologists who have reached the conclusion that we are created by God in his image."
> —Dr. Johanna Budwig

Ideal Foliar Feeding Applications Guidelines	
Time of Day to Apply	Early morning before 9:00 a.m. Late evening after 6:00 p.m.
Temperature	65° - 85° Fahrenheit, 70° ideal
Wind speed	Less than 5 mph (A plant can detect a small change in carbon dioxide in air, even blowing on them can close stomata.)

Just One Foliar Feeding Benefits Wheatgrass

For further clarification, when you mist your sprouting seeds with the water and sea solids fertilizer spray in the beginning sprouting stages, you are certainly both fertilizing and hydrating them. However, the *larger* surface area *only* located on the grass *leaves* have *both* the absorbent epidermis and stomata valves which do a fantastic job of taking in this extra liquid nutrition. Increased surface area on the leaves themselves means increased nutrient absorption possibilities.

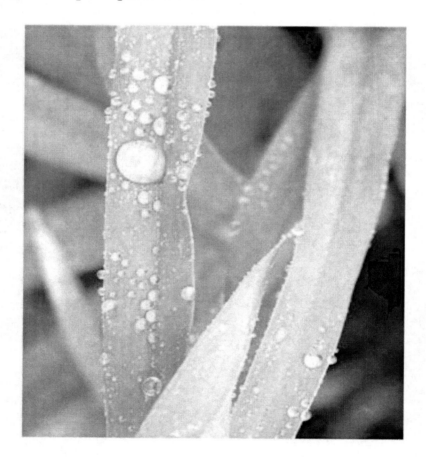

You can foliar feed with the water and sea solids fertilizer, when *not* watering with a fine mist sprayer as yes indeed those moistened leaves of wheatgrass will be able to take in the nutrition from larger droplets of hydration. **However, the *tinier* and more *numerous* the droplets on the surface of the leaves, the better nutrient absorption.** Therefore, the easy to use *fine* mist sprayer is the *ideal* foliar feeding tool.

The nutritious mist can easily be directed to make contact and penetrate *all* the blades of grass from a variety of different directions and angles.

> **"Minerals are the foundation for life, even if many have still to be researched and understood."**
> —*Charles Walters*

Additionally, only *one* foliar feeding will benefit your growing wheatgrass. In fact, just one or two foliar feedings can meet the entire desire of the plant for many minerals and trace elements, as amounts required are very small. Taking that into consideration and understanding how the sea solids fertilizer not only nourishes but also protects and strengthens the wheatgrass, my preference is 2 - 3 foliar feedings during the growing cycle.

Which Days to Foliar Feed?

There is no "set in stone" foliar feeding schedule. **Foliar feeding can really be done at any time**, but for *optimum* results, do follow the Ideal Foliar Feeding Applications Guidelines chart located a few pages back.

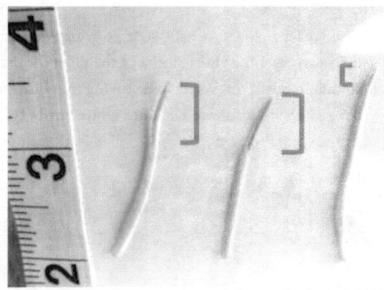

Miniature wheatgrass leaves emerge from their protective sheath (coleoptile) when sprouts are 1 - 2 inches tall.

When it comes to picking the *days* to foliar feed your wheatgrass, the following foliar feeding guidelines work quite well.

> **"From when sprouts are turning into grass leaves (about 1 - 2 inches tall) and up until harvest, you can provide 2 - 3 foliar feedings, which is plenty."**

You can give that *first* true *foliar* feeding as soon as the wheatgrass leaves begin to emerge from the sprouts—about when you permanently remove the growing cover and the grass is "out of the starting gate."

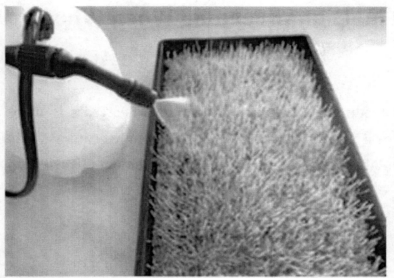

Apply first foliar feeding when grass leaves begin to emerge.

"Go ahead and provide the second foliar feeding about 3 - 4 days after the first foliar feed. And you can apply the *final* foliar feeding 3 - 4 days after the second foliar feed."

You can foliar feed on those days when you are not watering the soil because it is already plenty moist. For best results, you can foliar spray in the morning or evening as per the Ideal Foliar Feeding Applications Guidelines chart recommendations.

Spray Final Foliar Feeding When Wheatgrass Leaf Has Larger Surface Area

The third foliar feeding will be given when the wheatgrass is more fully grown and *broad* leafed with a nice larger surface area. If your wheatgrass wants these perfectly balanced, bioavailable liquid minerals and trace elements, it will happily take them in from the surface of its leaves.

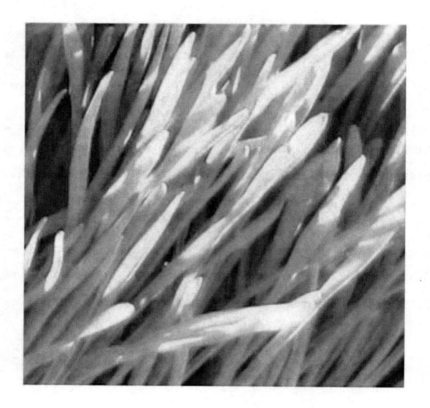

And let's say its nutritional desires are *already* nicely met; well, the sea solids fertilizer will still further support the successful growth of your plant. You really can't lose!

As a point of interest, I have watered with the sea solids solution every day up until the leaf stage, then hydrated and fed the wheatgrass henceforth with both the foliar spray method *and* watering can method using the sea solids and water solution. The wheatgrass was hydrated with the sea solids and water recipe every single day. No negative effects were shown by the wheatgrass, as wheatgrass does quite well in a highly saline growing environment.

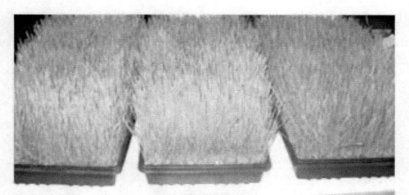

Wheatgrass hydrated frequently and solely with water and SEA-90 sea mineral solids solution flourishes.

Finally, keep in mind, foliar feeding is an *optional* added nutrient uptake opportunity and a way to *further* support your crop. If you choose to foliar feed, a little goes a long way with this fantastic fertilizing sea spray.

Side note: If you choose to fertilize, you can certainly incorporate and experiment with your other favorite fertilizers along with the sea solids (if you use them). I focus on the sea solids fertilizing solution because of its outstanding results. I know you will grow *exceptionally* nutritious wheatgrass with its inclusion. **And I want *each one* of the minerals and trace elements found in the ocean's potion**—multitudinous minerals and trace elements highly valuable to our wheatgrass and us.

What If I Want to Water With Only the Sprayer?

You can certainly choose to water your wheatgrass (from seed to harvest) *solely* with a *sprayer* applying the water and sea solids fertilizer solution. That's fine, your wheatgrass will also turn out beautiful this way too. Just make sure to apply enough water when those growing green blades are taller and thirstier.

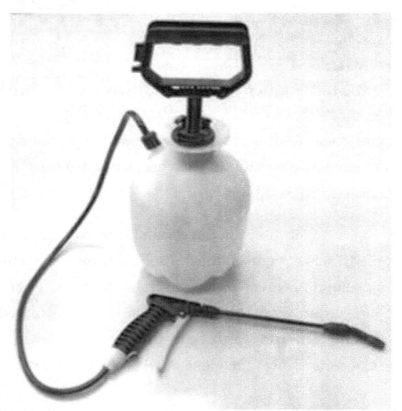

FloMaster one gallon sprayer works well and is BPA free.

I have presented the watering methods I have found to be the most successful, but you can certainly vary your approach. You can experiment with the amount and timing of foliar feedings you choose to apply, as well as try out different salinity levels. Your wheatgrass will communicate to you visually just how pleased it is with your choices.

Again, feel free to try out other soil fertilizers for your wheatgrass, as it is always interesting to experiment. Make sure the other selected fertilizer can be absorbed by the wheatgrass. The wheatgrass is grown and harvested too quickly for soil microorganisms to fully digest non-soluble minerals and make them available for the plant.

Overall, "capturing" the essence of the ocean in the sea solids, and nourishing your wheatgrass with them, is an excellent way to go as they are second to none. Out of all the plants, wheatgrass is the only plant known to absorb 90 plus elements. SEA-90 life supporting and fortifying sea solids provide a *full* feast of minerals and trace elements for the wheatgrass—a true nutrient uptake expert.

Simple Recipe for Making Mineral Rich Liquid Fertilizer

It is simple to make a SEA-90 sea solids and water solution for *both* soil fertilization and foliar feeding your wheatgrass. If you cannot obtain the SEA-90 sea solids garden fertilizer which is the best choice and that is *superb* for wheatgrass growing, you can use an ocean harvested sea salt as explained below.

You are certainly welcome to experiment with different salinity levels, but the below recipe works quite well for wheatgrass. **Do not use refined, mineral and trace element depleted salt.**

Fertilizer Recipe

Mix 1 Gallon of Water With 1 Teaspoon SEA-90 Sea Solids

(Or other ocean harvested sea salt with full spectrum of minerals and trace elements)

Recommended Ocean Based Fertilizers

1. SEA-90 Sea Solids at SeaAgri.com – Perfect for wheatgrass

2. Well selected non-refined sea salt harvested from fresh seawater that best preserves the full spectrum of minerals and trace elements

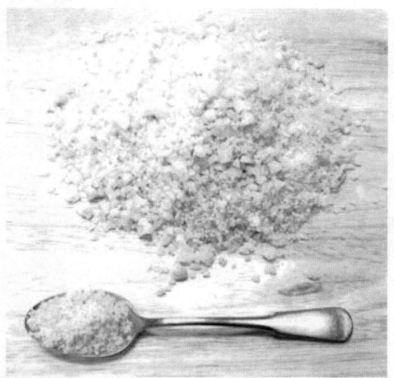

SEA-90 sea solids are a superior natural and sustainable fertilizer.

"Stir the SEA-90 sea solids and water together until the grains dissolve—the *larger* particles from the grains *may* require several hours or overnight to dissolve—especially if using a larger salty grain like SEA-90 sea solids.

With SEA-90 sea solids, any residue still existing is both non-liquefying rock dust and crystals too large to quickly liquefy."

"It is axiomatic that if the minerals are missing, the hope for excellent health and genetics is in vain....

"Phosphate is a necessary element for energy molecules associated with the Krebs cycle. Magnesium is associated with over 300 enzymatic reactions....

"There are 92 non-radioactive elements. Do they all have a role? In about 400 years we will know, if the present rate of discovery is continued....

"We know about zinc and some 200 enzyme processes the element accounts for. We know about copper and healthy blood cells. We know manganese is necessary for conception. We know boron is associated with parathyroid gland function.

"And we know about a few others, but mostly the best settled science is still in the dark about what the cow has been trying to tell us."

—Charles Walters
Grass - the Forgiveness of Nature

Chapter 8: How to Sprout Seeds First, Before "Planting" (Method Two)

"Stay close to nature and its eternal laws will protect you."

–Dr. Max Gerson

Sprouting Seeds Before Planting is Not Necessary

Some people like to *sprout* their wheat seeds *before* planting them in the soil. You are certainly welcome to do this extra sprouting step, if you feel it will help your wheatgrass yield.

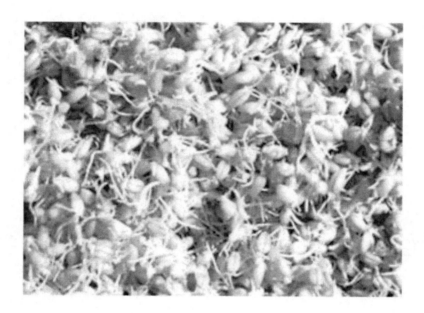

I have found sprouting my grains (after soaking them) to obtain that 1/4 – 1/2 inch sprout on my wheat seeds, and then to plant them, to be an unnecessary and more time consuming step. I seek simplicity when growing wheatgrass.

Personally, I simply rinse the seeds, soak the seeds, rinse again, and then plant them. I do not sprout them for an additional day before I plant them. I have not found that sprouting step to increase my yield or health of the wheatgrass.

However, if you would like to take the extra step of sprouting your seeds *before you plant* them, that is fine. You may enjoy this step or find it of value.

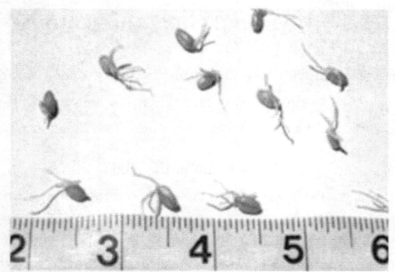

Seeds are ready to plant when their sprouts are between 1/4 – 1/2 inch long.

Following are the sprouting seeds before planting instructions. Once again, I will teach you this step, but it *is not necessary* to produce a beautiful yield of wheatgrass.

Sprouting Seeds Beginning Steps

First, rinse your seeds well with lukewarm water. About 30 seconds worth of rinsing is good. As mentioned earlier, rinsing your seeds first will help wash off microorganisms that can be on the surface of the seed, which can lead to increased mold.

Second, soak your seeds from 8 - 12 hours in the colder winter, or 6 - 8 hours in the warmer temperatures, when the benefits of soaking occur at a more rapid pace.

Place your pre-rinsed seeds in the soaking bowl. Then, cover the seeds with lukewarm water. You want 3 times as much water as seeds in your bowl. So, when I soak 1 1/2 cups of wheatgrass seeds in water, I soak them in 4 1/2 cups of water. The seeds soak up a lot of the water, so you want to make sure you have plenty of it. Make sure your bowl is large enough to accommodate the larger size of sprouted seeds.

Also, **add 1 teaspoon of SEA-90 sea solids to the water and seeds** and stir everything together for a few seconds until sea solids are dissolved.

Third, after the soaking stage is complete, rinse off those pre-soaked seeds once more with lukewarm water. A 15 - 30 seconds or so rinse is fine:
1. Rinse
2. Soak
3. Rinse

Rinse Sprouting Wheat Seeds Two Times Per Day

Place previously soaked and then strained seeds in a bowl or a strainer. (A strainer makes them very easy to later rinse by just rinsing them while in the strainer, recovering, and then setting the strainer on a plate to catch their drainage.)

Continuing with the bowl method, cover the seeds with a moist towel or piece of plastic on top. Both a cloth towel and a plastic wrap work well, though I prefer the extra 'breathability" of the cloth towel. This covering will help keep the grains moist during the sprouting stage. The sprouting process will now begin.

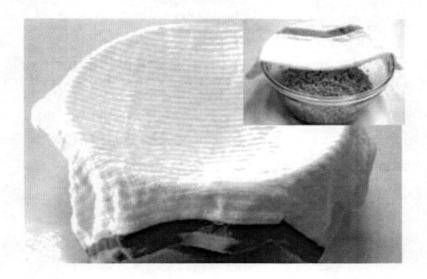

Next, about 8 to 12 hours later, you will give your sprouting seeds their first rinse. **Rinse your sprouting seeds with clean lukewarm water 2 - 3 times per day.** You can simply use your kitchen faucet to put clean water into the bowl, swoosh seeds around in the water, and then drain. A single rinse is just fine.

Or, pour the seeds into a colander or strainer and rinse under the faucet. A 30 second rinse in lukewarm water is fine. You can rinse any way you prefer. What is important is that the seeds are rehydrated through this process. This rinse also serves as a nice cleansing. Make sure seeds are well drained, then place back in bowl, if they had been removed, and cover with the plastic wrap or a wet towel again. The rinsed and drained wheat seeds are then to continue their sprouting.

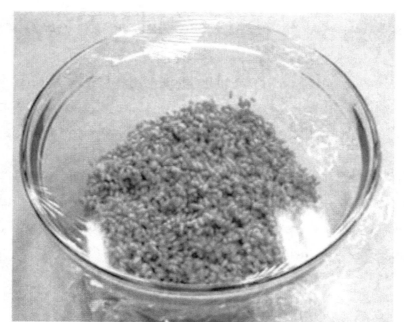

**Rinse 2 – 3 times per day. A morning and evening rinse is good;
or a morning, noon, and evening rinse works well too.**

Additionally, if you prefer, you can sprout your seeds in a sprouting jar or a sprouting bag. What is important is that the sprouting seeds are rinsed off with clean water 2 – 3 times per day and that the water is then drained from the seeds.

Transplant Seeds After Sprouts Emerge

First the tiny white rootlets emerge, then shortly afterwards the beginnings of the wheatgrass blades peek out and make their debut—*both* sprouting out from the same end of the wheat seed.

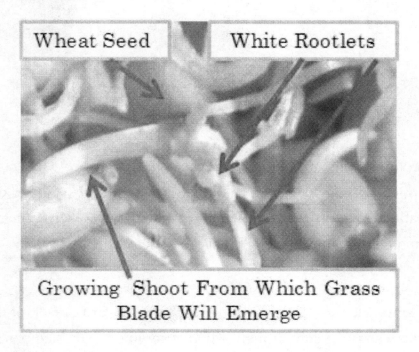

When you see that the little sprouts have emerged from the seeds and are about 1/4 – 1/2 inch long, the sprouted wheat seeds are ready to be transplanted. **It only takes 24 – 48 hours for the moistened seeds in your sprouting container to shoot forth 1/4 – 1/2 inch long sprouts.**

What if you get busy and do not have time to plant your sprouted grains and those sprouts are now longer than 1/4 – 1/2 inch long? That's fine, just go ahead and plant them with those longer sprouts.

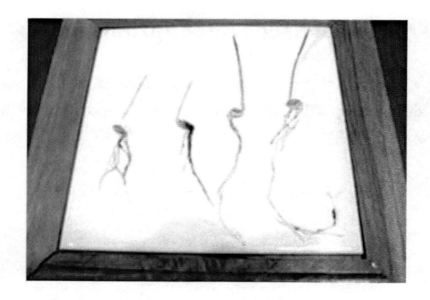

Once these sprouted seeds are placed atop the soil in your growing tray, their porous and tubular rootlets will quickly begin to burrow down into the soil and disappear from view. They instinctively proceed southbound, navigating away from the light and steadfastly maneuvering into the dark soil to obtain their nutrients, like a feeding earthworm.

On the other hand, the young blades innately grow upwards reaching for the golden sunlight. There is a sense of contentment when observing the miraculous blades of grass and the hungry and thirsty rootlets each charting their own perfect pre-programmed course for the proliferation of the plant.

Place Sprouts Atop Soil, Water, and Cover Sprouts

Place those sprouted grains right onto the surface of your soil and then spread them out evenly.

Next, water them with about 2 cups of the water and sea solids solution.

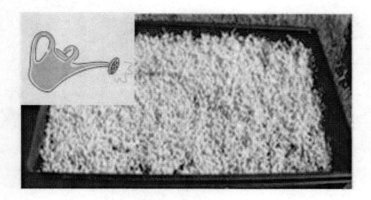

You want to water enough to moisten not only the sprouted seeds, but also the soil directly beneath them. The little roots like to expand in moist soil. You can water the seeds initially with a watering can or mister.

Again, you do not *need* to add sea solids to your water. I grew many batches of wheatgrass without it—or any fertilizer. However, my "green thumb" improved greatly and my wheatgrass was far more vibrant, through adding sea solids to the water. Also, sea solids are the best for using in the soaking step, but you *can* use another unrefined sea salt. For the main fertilizing though, you will receive the best harvest with SEA-90 sea solids.

Finally, place your cover over those sprouts until the wheatgrass is 1 – 2 inches tall.

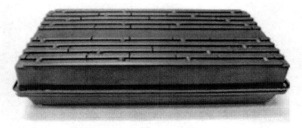

Mist the sprouts with the water and sea solids solution about once per day during the covered sprouting stage, as explained in Chapter 6. You want enough water to moisten the sprouts and the soil. Proceed taking care of this *pre-sprouted* wheatgrass the same as wheatgrass that was *not* pre-sprouted—as was described in Chapter 6.

"Remember, grass is the only vegetation on the face of the earth that will healthfully support an animal from birth to a prime old age. I am surprised that more attention has not been given to this kind of vegetation as a food for human beings."

—Dr. G.H. Earp-Thomas
*World Expert on Grass and
Soil Analyzation*

Chapter 9: Troubleshooting Strategies and How to Reduce Mold (Method Three and Four)

"In *Eco-Farm, An Acres U.S.A. Primer*, it was settled without fear of contradiction that plants in touch with balanced nutrition, with a full variety of trace minerals, create their own hormone and enzyme potentials and therefore protect themselves against bacterial, fungal, viral and insect attack. Much the same is true for human beings...."

—Charles Walters
Fertility From the Ocean Deep

Mold and Sprouting Problems

When I first started growing wheatgrass, before using the nourishing sea solids and water mixture and learning how to best grow wheatgrass, I struggled for years with periodic mold and inconsistent germination rates. I hope the following growing challenges and tips will help you.

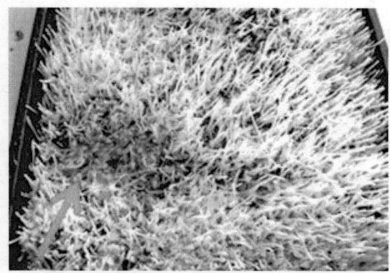

Mold sets in when germination falters.

I will share my wheatgrass growing challenges to help you realize that if I can learn how to successfully grow wheatgrass, you certainly can too. If you have experienced the same disappointing wheatgrass growing results, seeing my sad looking wheatgrass might help you feel less discouraged. Or at the very least, these pictures will give you a good laugh!

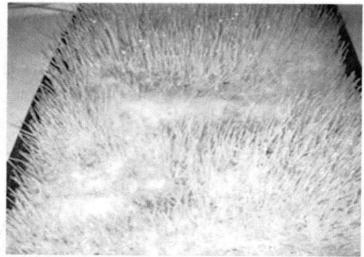
White cotton-like mold has overtaken wheatgrass tray.

Here are some helpful wheatgrass growing facts:

- *Healthy* seeds and plants are better able to resist disease and fight off pathogens
- When something is wrong or out of balance with wheatgrass, plant becomes perfect prey for pathogens, and for mold to take over
- Mold-ridden wheatgrass is not fit to be consumed
- Pathogens thrive in anaerobic, low oxygen conditions
- Beneficial organisms thrive with more oxygen, aerobic conditions
- With a little growing mold, watering will wash it away—like a good cleansing rain
- Placing wheatgrass outside, even temporarily, decreases mold challenges—feel free to water with outdoor hose sprayer

Easily Remove Mold or Fungus Affecting Small Areas

Here is another example of a wheatgrass growing problem I experienced. Sometimes, a small patch of seeds would not sprout and then mold would set in. To save the harvest, you can take a spoon or other tool and scoop away the moldy area. This step definitely helps prevent the mold from spreading and allows you to save the wheatgrass harvest.

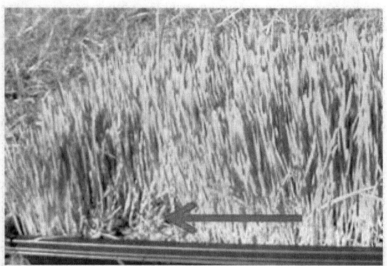

**Mold sets in when seeds do not germinate in certain areas
of your wheatgrass tray.**

> **"If you still see a little grayish-white, cotton-like mold at the base
> of your wheatgrass, you can cut *above* the mold when harvesting
> and rinse it well to avoid consuming it."**

As mentioned, before I started using the fortifying and protective sea solids solution, my growing wheatgrass seeds were much more susceptible to mold and had a lower germination rate.

Before I included the sea solids along with the pre-soaking seeds and into their "diet," my wheatgrass seeds and growing wheatgrass would be much more sensitive to *non-perfection* in their growing habitat. Soaking the seeds and fertilizing with the sea solids and water solution, resulted in a far hardier wheatgrass crop with a higher yield.

189

"Before growing a new batch of wheatgrass, it's best to make sure the trays from the last batch are clean and have no mold on them. Soap and water works nicely to clean the trays."

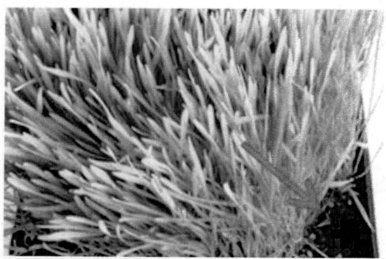

Moldy wheatgrass in corner is removed to help prevent mold from spreading to entire batch of wheatgrass.

Sprouting Seeds Need Ample Water

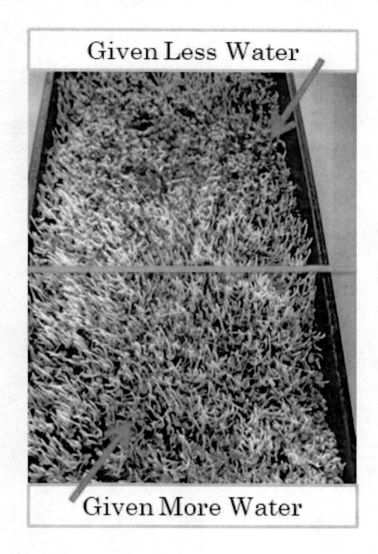

Given Less Water

Given More Water

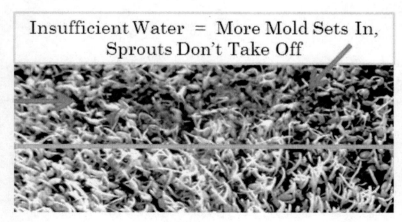

Insufficient Water = More Mold Sets In, Sprouts Don't Take Off

You can also *under* water your sprouting seeds. The wheat seeds in the top half of the two photos, received *less* water than those in the bottom half. The top half was lightly sprayed, and water did not reach the soil directly beneath the seeds. The wheat seeds in the bottom half of the pictures received ample water.

With insufficient water, the germination faltered and more mold developed. Soaking *and* fertilizing wheatgrass with the sea solids and water solution *decreases* seed sensitivity to non-ideal growing conditions, and *increases* disease resistance of seeds.

Rinse Seeds Before Soaking for Better Growing Results

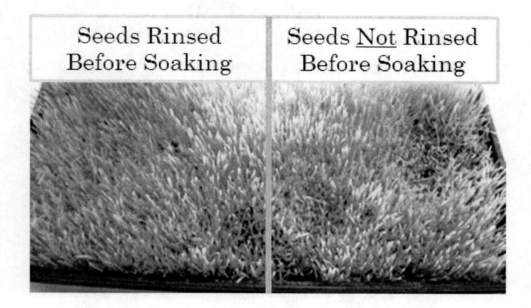

There are microorganisms that live on the surface of the seed and actually under the surface of the seed too. Rinsing the outside of your seeds will reduce these microorganisms that can contribute to mold on your wheatgrass and to poor growth.

The fungal pathogens found in the soil can also rot (decompose) the seed before it sprouts.

Watering Amount and Pre-Rinsing Seed Affects Germination

Problems with mold can also result from *over* watering, as the following pictures show.

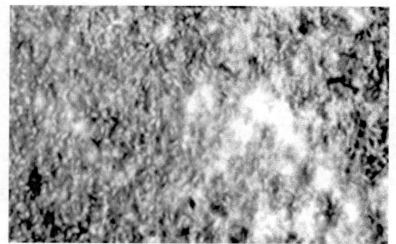

Mold can set in when wheatgrass is over watered.

Additionally, rinsing the seeds with lukewarm water *before* soaking them is a very beneficial step. If the pre-rinsing of wheat seeds step is skipped, incorporating *anti-bacterial* sea solids usage in wheatgrass watering will also help counter a propensity for mold. I always pre-rinse the seeds, as I like knowing I am helping to rinse off any potential disease-causing fungi and bacteria on the surface of the seed. This rinsing step is a simple and effective way to increase the success of your wheatgrass growing.

Once the wheatgrass seeds show signs of difficulty in sprouting, weakness and vulnerability, there are plenty of microscopic invaders ready to assist in decomposing them—which is nature's way. *Healthier* seeds and their *healthier* wheatgrass will not beckon the decomposers to begin their work—ensuring the hardiest crops flourish for our nutritional enjoyment.

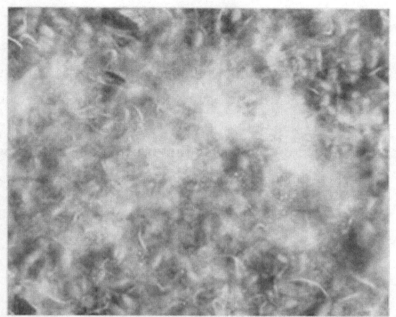

Close-up of over watered seeds, mold has overtaken them.

These pictures on poor wheatgrass growth were taken prior to incorporating sea solids usage and fine tuning the growing process. I hope they are beneficial in helping you see and understand that growing wheatgrass may not always work out perfectly. But fortunately, by following the instructions in this *How to Grow Glorious Wheatgrass at Home Tutorial*, you will find your wheatgrass growing "green thumb" too!

How to Eliminate Fruit Flies

Yes, those bothersome fruit flies can take a liking to wheatgrass. Fruit flies can hitchhike in on fruits and vegetables that you have purchased. If some over-ripened fruit in your kitchen has attracted these quickly multiplying fruit flies to lay their eggs upon them, they will hatch and then feed on the fermenting fruit. The fruit flies prefer the alcohol content and yeast in fermenting or rotting foods. Maybe their poor flying abilities are an indication of their diet!

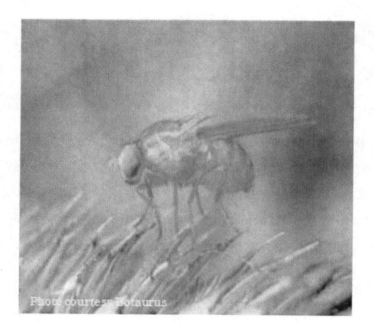

Next thing you know, these pesky fruit flies will grow in number and notice your growing wheatgrass. They can then decide to land on your wheatgrass and stay awhile.

> **"Fruit flies can lay more than 500 eggs at a time, and have a life cycle of about 10 – 18 days."**

If this becomes a problem with the fruit flies and you want to get rid of them, here are some steps you can take:

- Do your best to toss any over-ripened fruit on your counter to prevent their arrival. By removing any over-ripened foods they can feed on, they will shortly be gone.

• If there are lots of fruit flies on your tray of wheatgrass, quickly cover your tray with a towel to capture them. Then, take the tray outside, lift towel and release them. If possible, you can keep your trays of wheatgrass outside for a few days, until the inside fruit fly population decreases. Make sure none are remaining on wheatgrass when you bring tray back inside.

• You can also try a vacuum cleaner, but many will get away.

• Preventing them in the first place is easiest.

Cover Seeds With Light Layer of Soil for Mold Reduction Strategy (Method Three)

If you are struggling with mold, or would like to attempt another growing method, you can certainly grow your wheatgrass seeds with a light layer of soil over them. You may notice you have less mold with this growing strategy.

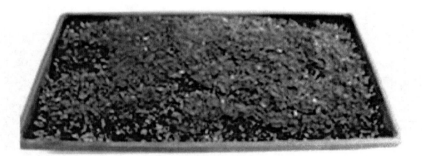

If you try growing your wheatgrass this way, and since you will be adding additional soil on top of your seeds, you can start with less *original* soil in your growing tray.

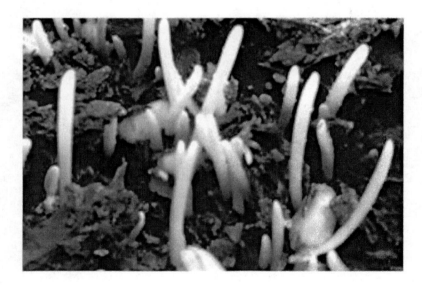

Since you have the soil serving as the perfect wheatgrass cover, you will *not* need to place a plastic cover over the seeds while they are sprouting.

> **"You may find the "breathable" and protective soil to be the perfect cover for your wheatgrass, as it is hard to beat Mother Nature."**

To continue, the wheatgrass will emerge through the soft soil, many times lifting up the soil with it. Now, as you water, some of the soil will be rinsed down below the base of the wheatgrass blades. But at harvest time, some unwanted soil on your wheatgrass blades may still remain.

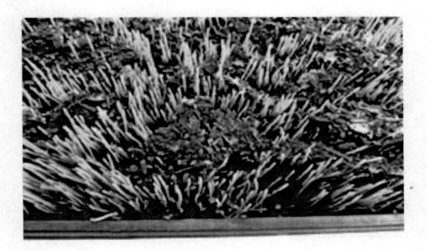

If at harvesting time, there is still unwanted soil atop your wheatgrass, or lodged in between the blades, you may choose to water with a little more force.

Before Harvest, Rinse Off Soil with a
Little Stronger Force

If you need to rinse away soil, you can try using a sprayer on your sink faucet, or even a water sprayer outside. Go ahead and separate the blades of grass with your hand to rinse more thoroughly between the blades.

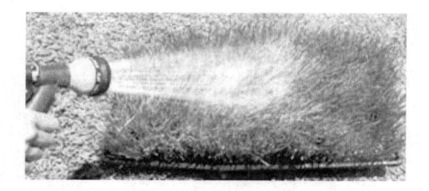

When you use a stronger sprayer and thus apply more water, be sure your tray of wheatgrass has adequate drainage. When spraying outside, take off the bottom tray with no holes. This will allow plenty of good drainage. If the weather is right, you can certainly continue growing it outside. Or after draining well, replace the bottom tray with no holes and set it back inside on your counters.

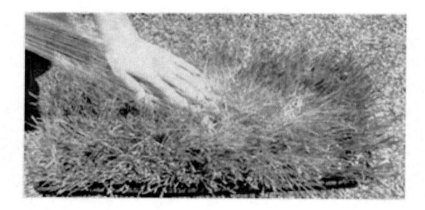

Side note: Outdoor water spraying, then keeping tray outdoors in natural elements, is also a great strategy for addressing mold that has accumulated at the base of your wheatgrass.

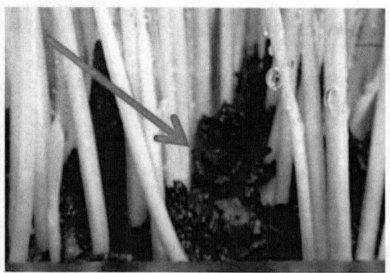

Soil is lodged at base of wheatgrass.

Even when choosing an extra rinsing method, at harvesting time some soil may *still* be lodged in between the base of the grass stems. You can then either cut your wheatgrass *above* the soil line, or actually cut through this lodged soil and make sure to rinse it well.

The reason this method is not as popular is because the top added layer of soil is mixed in amongst those growing blades of wheatgrass, thus it can be more difficult to rinse off after harvesting. Keep in mind, a *thinner* layer of that added top soil, will certainly make the rinsing step much easier. Following are the instructions to grow the wheatgrass with a light layer of soil over the wheat seeds....

Simple Growing Instructions for Seeds Covered with Soil

If you choose to grow your wheatgrass with soil over the seeds, growing instructions are really about identical to the regular instructions. Again, you do not need to use a plastic cover, since the soil serves as the cover.

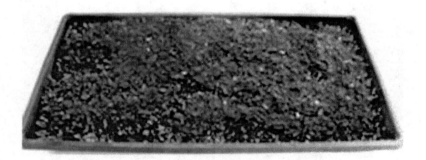

Use the same amount of seeds mentioned earlier and pre-treat (rinse and soak) them the same way. Instructions are:

1. Place your pre-treated seeds atop your bed of soil.

2. Place a light layer of soil on top of the seeds. About 2 cups of soil (you can vary the amount) to provide a *thin* layer of soil above your seeds.

3. Water with sea solids and water solution mentioned earlier in tutorial. When watering, you can always (each and every time you water) use this *select* fertilizing solution. You can also foliar feed as explained in Chapter 7.

4. The first time you water the soil and underlying seeds, use about 4 cups of water— enough to nicely moisten the top and bottom soil surrounding the seeds. A watering can or sprayer is fine.

5. 24 hours after initial watering, water again with either watering can or sprayer, enough to keep soil and seeds beneath moistened. You will not need as much water as initially used. Repeat this step every 24 hours until grass blades are about one inch high.

6. Once the baby blades of grass are over one inch high, go ahead and increase the amount of water they receive, as they are thirstier. A watering can works well.

7. From this point forward, water every day, or every other day as needed—like original watering instructions.

8. Enjoy your harvest!

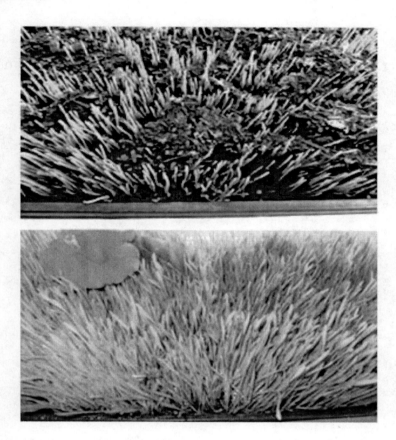

Plant Seeds On Top of Soil - With No Plastic Cover (Method Four)

Here is another option to grow your wheatgrass which you just may enjoy. This is another growing wheatgrass method if you are still struggling with mold, or would just like to just have fun experimenting.

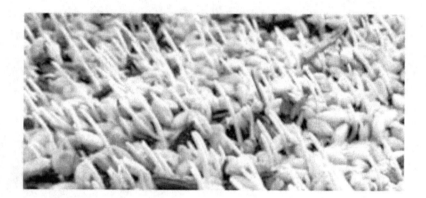

Simply place your growing seeds on top of your soil, as prior instructions explain. But, instead of placing a plastic tray as a cover, *there will be no cover*—allowing more air and its oxygen to reach your seeds. That's right, just "plant" the seeds without adding a cover and otherwise follow the same growing instructions in Chapter 6. Watering with about 2 cups of water after seeds have been "planted," should be good for your initial watering.

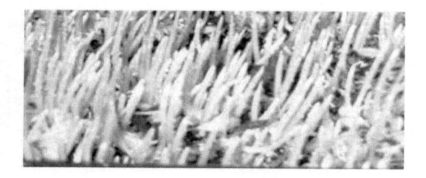

Keep in mind, since there is no cover on top of your seeds to help keep them moist, they will be more prone to drying out. You will have to be *extra vigilant* about keeping them moist. You will most likely need to water them at least 2 times per day, maybe more, depending on your growing environment.

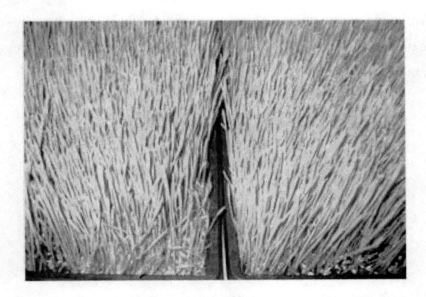

Again, the downside or challenge with this growing method is keeping the seeds moistened, as they are most particular during their sprouting stage. Additionally, you may find there is less of a germination rate because they are drying out.

Finally, the upside of this growing method is since you have no plastic cover on top of your wheatgrass, there is now increased air circulation with plenty of oxygen for your sprouts—thus less likelihood of mold.

Paper Towels are Not Necessary

I used to place paper towels on top of my wheatgrass seeds during their sprouting stage until they were about one inch tall, but for the sake of simplicity, I no longer use them as my sprouting cover.

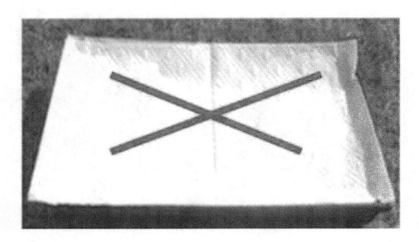

Bad bacteria flourish in environments with less oxygen, and higher oxygen levels support the good bacteria. These good bacteria in the soil support the sprouting seeds and also nourish their growth. I, therefore, started questioning just how "breathable" and necessary my moistened paper towels really were. I wondered if they were contributing to more mold.

Wanting to avoid having to use paper towels and certainly not wanting to use newspaper as a sprouting cover either, I substituted an inverted black plastic wheatgrass tray with the holes on top as the sprouting cover. This covering could be used over and over again, and the covering *with the holes* allowed for more oxygen to reach the sprouting seeds.

You can certainly use other items as a cover like an old t-shirt. Just make sure the cover you select keeps the moisture in, light out, and that it is "breathable," therefore allowing oxygen to reach the seeds and soil. Preferably, I would not place your cover of choice directly on top of the sprouting seeds. Place it up and over the edges of the wheatgrass tray so it does not rest directly upon the seeds.

How to Store Harvested Wheatgrass

If you will not be able to consume your entire batch of wheatgrass while in its peak state of health, feel free to store it. You have the option to completely harvest the *entire* wheatgrass tray once it hits the magic 7-inch mark.

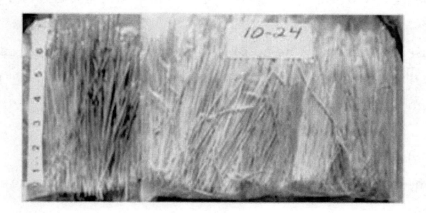

Simply cut all of your mature wheatgrass and store it in a plastic bag for later juicing. This way, you never have to worry about your wheatgrass starting to wilt because it has not been harvested when 7 - 10 inches tall. Plus, you eliminate the wheatgrass tray on your counter, thus freeing up your space.

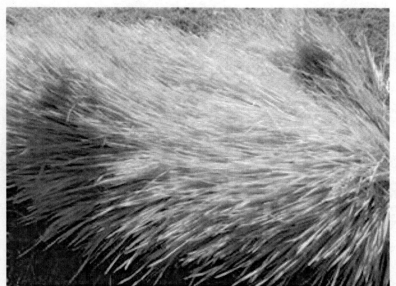

Grass loses its color, wilts, and falls over when past its harvesting time.

Is it as nutritious as cutting and then *immediately* juicing your wheatgrass? No, fresher wheatgrass is best. However, plenty of people prefer to harvest and store their wheatgrass in this manner and they still experience the profound benefits from drinking wheatgrass juice:

- You will be surprised how fresh it still tastes this way
- Stored wheatgrass in sealed plastic bag or container will stay good for one week in refrigerator
- Do not rinse wheatgrass before putting it in refrigerator for storage, as it will quicken the decomposing process like with other fruits and vegetables (rinse it right before you juice it later)
- Wheatgrass juice starts going bad within 30 minutes
- Best to drink *right after* juicing for optimum nutrition
- Discard wheatgrass juice if not used right away, as at it will be totally spoiled in about 12 hours

"Nature cures, but she needs an opportunity, and opportunity means following the Laws of Nature. Nature cleanses and purifies the body very slowly. You must use good foods consistently over a period of time to expect some changes. Wonder drugs, although offering speedy relief, seldom cure, and those immediate reliefs are brothers to silent partners such as side effects and drug accumulations."

—Charles Kellogg
The Soils That Support Us

Chapter 10: How to Make a Soil Sifter

"Unfortunately, no machine can show what nourishment may be missing from our ailing body and no group of savants, no matter how learned, can more than guess what our sick body lacks. And as this country bears the disgraceful reputation of being the 'sickest civilized nation on earth' those guesses in the past, must have been faulty."

—Ann Wigmore
Why Suffer? The Answer? Wheatgrass God's Manna

Make a Soil Sifter if Needed

Sometimes *unknowingly*, you may purchase soil with too much debris like little rocks or bark. You may also have compost or other soil at home with unwanted debris. Such soil will need to be filtered for more successful wheatgrass growing. If you are using soil without the larger matter, you can skip this sifting step.

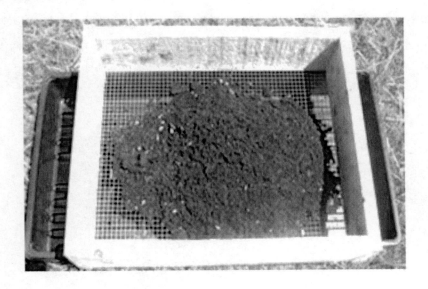

You can simply make a soil sifter at home, as I will show you. Or, you can buy one.

Perhaps, showing you how to make a soil sifter might spark some ideas for you. You can create a different sifter most suited for your particular wheatgrass growing needs.

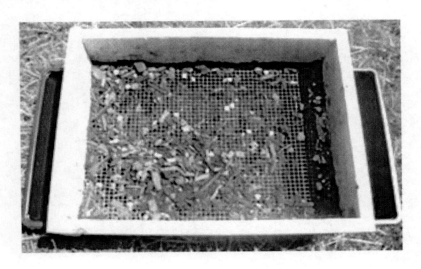

To sift your soil, place the sifter over the tray and shake the soil so it will work its way through to the bottom tray, leaving the larger items behind. You can also gently set filter on top of tray and use your hand or a tool to spread the soil around and rub it over the screen to work it through. Feel free to use your own filtering method.

You can buy all the materials for making a soil sifter at your local home improvement store. They may even cut the wood to the dimensions you request. Again, if you need a soil sifter, it may be easier for you to just buy one. But if you like to make things, I will show you how easy it is. You probably know a great way to make one too. This is just what worked for me.

Soil Sifter 12" X 15" Supplies & Directions

Gather the following supplies, or adapt the supplies to your situation:

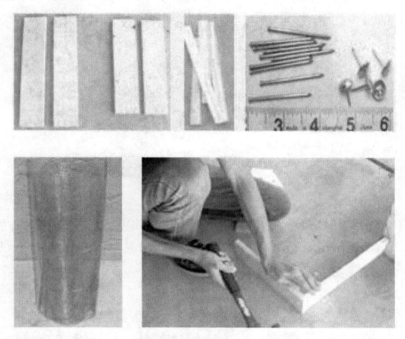

• 2 pieces wood 3 1/4" wide, 14" long, 5/8" thick

• 2 pieces wood 3 1/4" wide, 12" long, 5/8" thick

• 2 pieces wooden half-round molding strips 12" long, 5/8" wide

• 2 pieces wood strips 14" long, 5/8" wide

• 1 3/4" finishing nails (the real narrow ones with no wide flat top)

• 7/16" common nails or tacks, tack with wide flatter head was selected to hold down chicken wire

• 1/4" square chicken wire perfectly filters wheatgrass growing soil (might have to buy big role)

Nail together 4 larger pieces (two 12" long pieces and two 14" pieces) of wood end to end to form a rectangle. 14" pieces were nailed to *inside* ends of 12" pieces, as shown in photo. Hammer in narrow nails in direction of red arrows as shown in picture.

When nailing wooden ends together, place sifter against a supportive fixture.

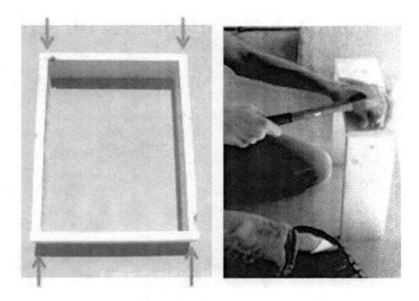

Unroll the chicken wire and place on a flat surface. Then, place your wooden rectangular frame on top of the filtering wire. Next, trace around the frame onto the wire with a crayon or chalk. The dimension will about 12" X 15".

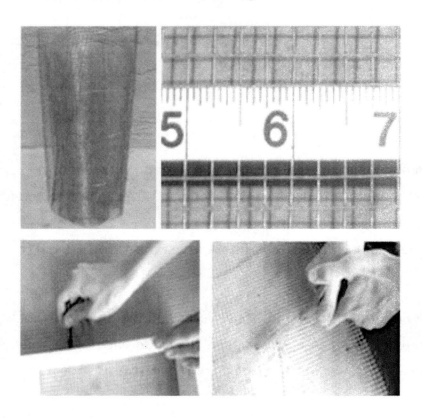

After you have traced, cut slightly *inside* the tracing marks as shown in the photo. An old pair of scissors works fine to cut this wire.

Place cut filtering wire on top of wooden frame, either side is fine. Nail in enough tacks to properly secure wire to wooden frame edging. Wide head of tacks will help hold and secure wire down.

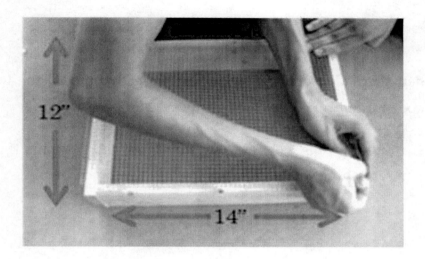

Alright, cut chicken wire, or filter, is now attached to wooden edging by tacks.

Here is what the soil sifter looks like with the filtering wire tacked on.

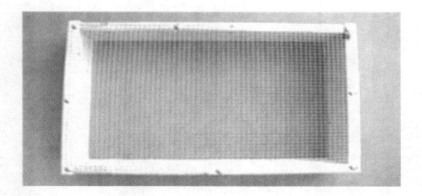

Next, place *flat* side of narrow half-round strips on top of surface of tacks, and nail together using narrow nails. The flat side of the 12" strip of wood sets atop 12" long edge of wooden frame. The flat side of the 14" strip of wood sets atop 14" long edge of wooden frame.

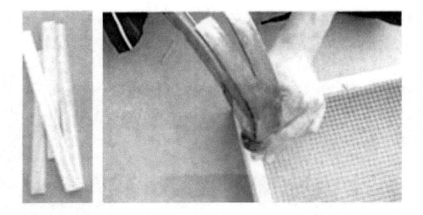

The four wooden strips that are 5/8" wide rest perfectly onto all the four wire sided edges of the wooden frame.

This wooden strip additionally secures your wire filter and prevents the edges of the chicken wire from scratching you.

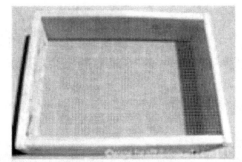

Completed sifter is upside down.

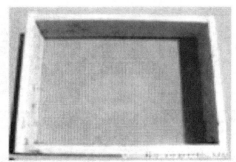

Completed sifter is right-side-up.

The soil and compost sifter is now complete. Next is a pictorial review on making this soil sifter.

Soil Sifter Pictorial Review

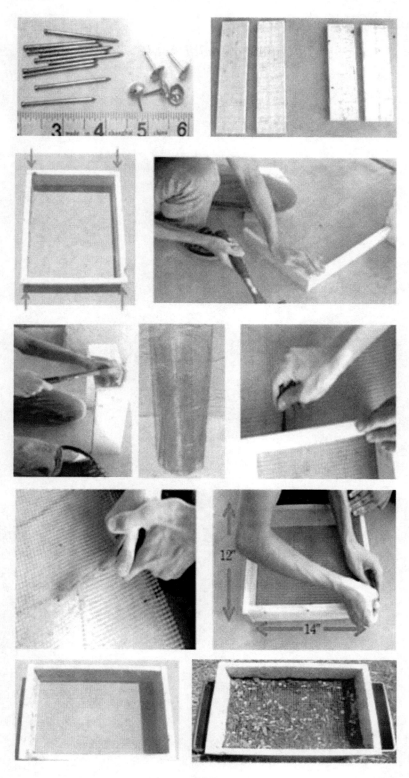

"So, remember that green grass is an incredibly good food for human consumption. If you ever get caught in a famine situation, just eat the grass—you'll do okay."

—William Campbell Douglass II, MD
The Raw Truth about Milk

Chapter 11: How to Obtain Wheat Seeds in Bulk and Store Properly

"After finding this quick-growing, vital grass to be of the richest in vitamins, minerals, and amino acids, I chose to work with it alone.

"It brought into my hands a simple, home-made food beverage which subsequent events suggested was capable of helping Mother Nature to mend shattered health and to extend the span of life."

—Ann Wigmore
Why Suffer, How I Overcame Illness and Pain Naturally

You Can Buy Wheat Seeds in Bulk

You may be able to obtain wheat seed in bulk locally. This bulk wheat seed may not be labeled for wheatgrass growing, but can still be *equally* good. See if you can buy a small batch of this non-designated wheat seed *before* buying a larger amount in bulk, to make sure you can grow wheatgrass successfully with it.

And as recommended earlier, before buying any non-designated wheat seed, you may want to *first* buy a *smaller* amount of wheatgrass growing seed from a supplier who sells top notch, specifically designated, wheatgrass seed—to help draw better growth comparisons.

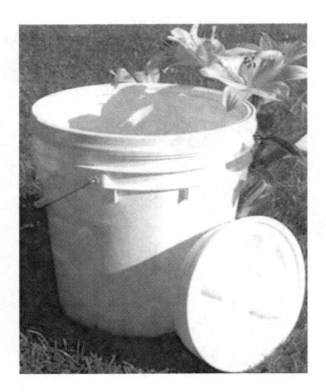

Here are options to locate wheat seeds in bulk for your wheatgrass growing:

- Check for a local co-op
- Check for local business that offers bread making classes, and that sells wheat grain
- Many churches and societies advise their members to store grain in bulk; they may have connections for you

- Amish Society
- Church of Jesus Christ of Latter-Day Saints
- Mennonite Church
- Seventh Day Adventist Church
- AzureStandard.com/getting-started – contact company for ordering guidelines and to find out drop point or delivery point of organic wheat seeds in your area
- Through HealthBanquet.com

> **"Our greatest weakness lies in giving up. The most certain way to succeed is always to try just one more time."**
> —*Thomas Edison*

Storage Tips for Wheat Seed

I buy my wheat seeds in bulk now, and prefer the hard white wheat seeds, as I use them for bread making too. Again, both Hard White Wheat Seed *and* Hard Red Wheat Seeds grow wonderful wheatgrass.

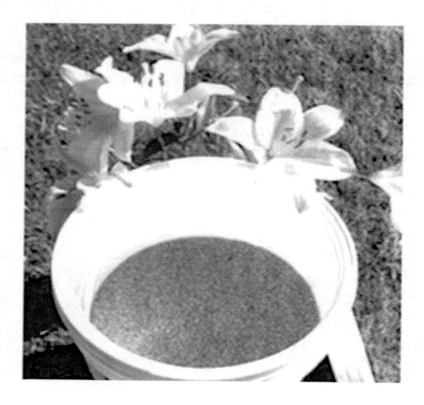

Here are proper storage tips for your seed:
- Best to keep wheat seeds dry, cool, and free from critters, to best preserve their quality
- You can store the precious seeds in a large 5 - 6.5 gallon bucket which stores about 50 lbs. of seed—this is the 6.5 gallon container I use
- This 12 inch in diameter bucket shown with the Gamma Seal Twistable Lid, keeps seeds dry and free from critters

> **"Wheat!... It is the sole agricultural product that has come down to us in the tombs of the early Egyptians....**
> **Wheat is the king of all food grains."**
> *—Dr. G.H. Earp-Thomas*

Wheat seed storage allows you to always have a great supply of wheat seeds on hand:

• Seeds will continue to sprout well for about 2 years, maybe longer if stored well

• I have used grain over a few years old and still grown wonderful wheatgrass

• For smaller amounts of wheatgrass seed, store in sealed container that keeps out moisture and critters—sealed plastic bag the seeds come in works out fine

Seed Storage Buckets Available in Different Sizes

Food grade storage buckets and Gamma Seal Lids are available for a low price at BaytecContainers.com:

- These buckets do come with the safety symbol that you see on the bucket
- These super heavy duty 90 mil plastic food grade buckets can be ordered in different sizes
- Keep in mind, you will use about 1 1/2 cup (about 3/4 pound) of seed per growing tray—producing about 12 - 15 ounces of wheatgrass juice

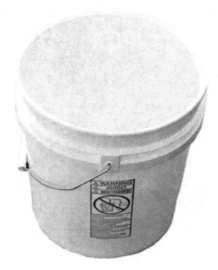

If seeds are stored in these airtight containers, they can last even longer for wheatgrass growing. Buckets with twist on lids are very good storage containers:

- 2 gallon buckets store about 14 lbs. of seed
- 3.5 gallon buckets store about 25 lbs. of seed
- 5 gallon buckets store about 35 lbs. of seed
- 6 gallon buckets store about 42 lbs. of seed

Place wheat seeds storage bucket in a nearby closet or pantry. If you buy or locate storage buckets, make sure they are food grade. You might be able to find free used food grade buckets at your local restaurant. And you may still want to purchase a Gamma Seal Lid which is available at BaytecContainers.com.

Gamma Seal Twist On Lid Works Well

You will love the easy *twist on* Gamma Seal Lid:

• Simply twist it off or spin it off to open, and twist back on or spin back on to close—works like a charm

• Quickly access your wheat seeds

• Gamma Seal Twist on lid comes with 1) Twist on lid and 2) A ring adapter to be attached to ordinary 12" in diameter pail or bucket (rubber mallet can be used to attach or hammer on ring to the lip of bucket)

• Lid then twists on smoothly and easily to this re-sealable ring adapter that is secured onto the lip of your bucket

• You can now preserve your bulk wheat seeds properly

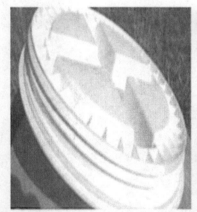 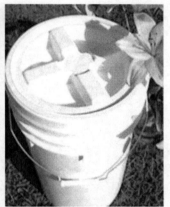

Bottom view of Gamma Seal twist on lid is on left, and lid is shown twisted securely in place onto top of bucket on right.

Storage Length of Wheat Seeds

Keep in mind if buying wheat seeds in bulk, viable wheat seeds are living organisms that are simply "resting" in their dormant state, waiting to be awakened. Even if properly stored, they slowly lose their vitality and decrease their germination rate over time. **If you buy good sprouting wheat seeds, they should maintain their germinating or sprouting ability for 2 years.** If the seeds are stored in a dry and cool location, they could last much longer.

"Grass is a balanced food containing a broad spectrum of high quality vegetable nutrition. It is a rainbow of food and at the end of the rainbow is the promise of golden health. Grass does not zoom you there with speed but carries you there gently on the magic carpet of endurance and delivers you with strength and longevity."

—Steve Meyerowitz
Wheatgrass - Nature's Finest Medicine

Chapter 12: Decorative Wheatgrass Centerpiece Examples

"Trace elements are a daily necessity in the diet of man and animals, as are vitamins, but it is apparent that trace elements, the biocatalysts, precede vitamins, and may actually cause their formation."

—Charles Walters
Grass – The Forgiveness of Nature

Wheatgrass Makes a Beautiful Centerpiece

Decorating with wheatgrass centerpieces is a wonderful way to add color, uniqueness, style, and liveliness, to a special occasion. Simply, basically follow the same wheatgrass growing instructions provided in this tutorial.

Plant more or less seeds, based on the density of wheatgrass you prefer. Increase or decrease the watering amount based on container size.

When it comes to a cover for your wheatgrass growing containers, you can place a towel over them. Remove the towel when sprouts are about one inch tall, and continue with the wheatgrass growing instructions in Chapter 6.

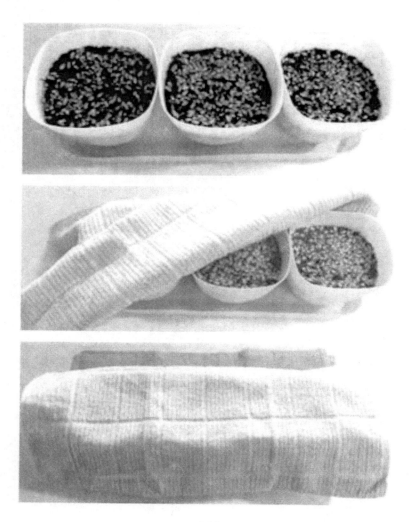

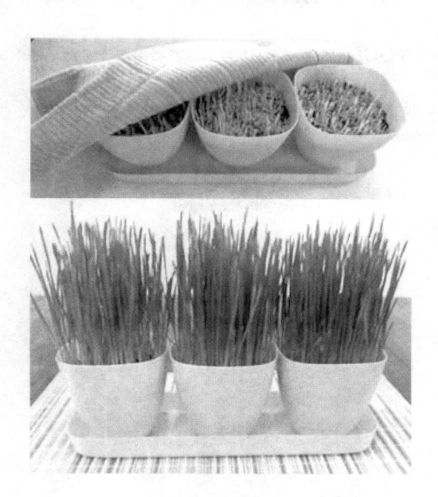

Choose Different Containers Based on Occasion

There are many ideas for beautiful wheatgrass decorations and centerpieces. Feel free to use your own imagination and creativity.

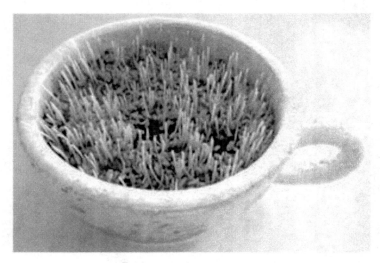

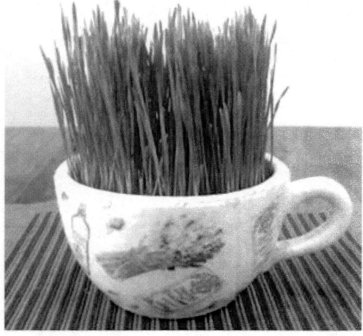

It is a wonderful way to bring the outdoors into your home, and to share a part of refreshing nature with your friends and loved ones. And, you can always consume the wheatgrass afterwards. In fact, you can even break off the grass blades at the dinner table and add them to your salads. Or, you can chew on a blade as an after-meal breath freshener. Let your personal taste guide you.

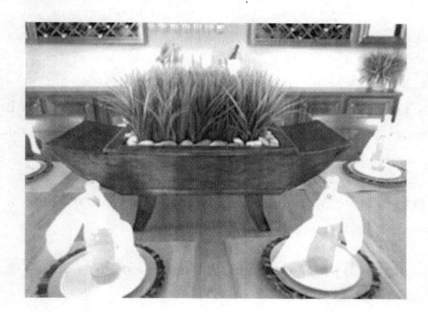

"My own experience exemplifies the miraculous ability of wheatgrass to fill deficiencies in the body and reverse the aging process. At fifty years of age I was ready for an early retirement. My hair was gray, I had a terrible case of colitis and other colon problems....

"In wheatgrass, raw foods, and exercise, I found what I feel is as close to the fountain of youth as we are going to get. Twenty-five years after my discovery, my hair has turned fully natural brown again. My weight has been a stable 119 (the same as it was in my youth), and my energy level is limitless....

"For the past ten years I have required an average of only four hours of sleep a night, and I haven't needed the services of a physician in years....

"I have more energy than I ever remember having as a child—I am no child at seventy-six. What I found can help you too."

—*Ann Wigmore*
The Wheatgrass Book

Chapter 13: Best Wheatgrass Growing Supplies and Resources

"A disease is to be cured naturally, by man's own powers; physicians merely help. Let your food be your medicine."

—Hippocrates

Wheatgrass Growing Supplies

Following are a few of the best wheatgrass growing supplies that are available through HealthBanquet.com at my Wheatgrass Growing Supplies store. These products will greatly help you successfully grow and juice wheatgrass at home.

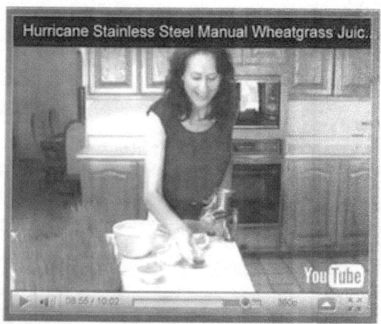

You Can View My How to Juice Wheatgrass with Hurricane Manual Juicer Video at YouTube or HealthBanquet.com

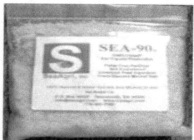

The SEA-90 sea solids are available at SeaAgri.com.

Wheatgrass Growing Kit With Hurricane Stainless Steel Manual Juicer

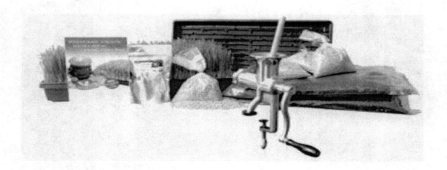

Wheatgrass Kit Includes:
Hurricane Manual Wheatgrass Juicer
5 21" X 11" X 2" growing trays
5 Lbs. organic wheatgrass seeds—Non-GMO seeds
• Yields 60 – 70 oz. of juice
Organic soil—enough for 5 – 6 trays of wheatgrass
Wheatgrass Book, Azomite Fertilizer
(Kit also available without juicer, or alternate juicers)
• Juicer attaches on counter or breadboard one and one half inches (1 1/2") wide or narrower
• Edge needs to jut out two inches (2") for juicer to attach
• Four inches (4") of vertical space below object it is attached to is required, for clamp-on device to fit

Organic Wheat Seeds, Pump Sprayers

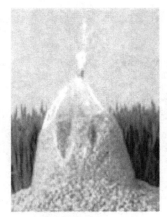

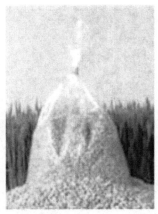

10 lb Bag Organic Hard
Red Wheat Grass Seeds

25 lb Bag Organic Hard
Red Wheat Grass Seeds

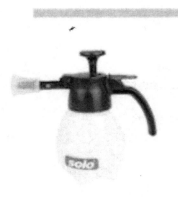

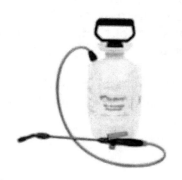

Solo 418 1-Liter
Pressure Sprayer

RL FloMaster 1
Gallon Sprayer

(Both sprayers are BPA free.)

Wheatgrass and Barley Grass Information

at HealthBanquet.com

- Ann Wigmore on Overcoming Illness with Wheatgrass
- Barley Grass Information
- Pastured Chickens Produce Brighter Orange Egg Yolks
- Chlorophyll in Wheatgrass
- Health Benefits of Wheatgrass Juice
- Natural Health Centers Serving Wheatgrass Juice
- Homemade Bread Made From Same Wheatgrass Seed
- Jesus Christ Reportedly Recommends Wheatgrass
- Medical Research on Wheatgrass
- Wheatgrass Growing Questions and Answers
- Wheatgrass Juice and Healthy Blood
- Wheatgrass Juice Testimonials
- Wheatgrass Juice Dosage Recommendations

Further Resources and Research

Wheatgrass and Barley Grass

Amici, M., L. Bonfili, M. Spina, V. Cecarini, I. Calzuola, V. Marsili, M. Angeletti, E. Fioretti, R. Tacconi, G.L. Gianfranceschi, A.M. Eleuteri. (2008). Wheat Sprout Extract Induces Changes on 20S Proteasomes Functionality, B*iochemie,* May; v.90(5): 790-801. http://www.sciencedirect.com/science/article/pii/S0300908407003239.

Bonfili, Laura, Manila Amici, Valentina Cecarini, Massimiliano Cuccioloni, Rosalia Tacconi, Mauro Angeletti, Evandro Fioretti, Jeffrey N. Keller, Anna Maria Eleuteri. Wheat Sprout Extract-Induced Apoptosis in Human Cancer Cells by Proteasomes Modulation. *Biochimi,* Sept; v(91): 1131-1144. http://www.sciencedirect.com/science/article/pii/S0300908409001588.

Calzuola, Isabella, Flavio Giavarini, Paola Sassi, Leonardo De Angelis, Gian Luigi Gianfranceschi, Valeria Marsili. (2005). Short Acidic Peptides Isolated From Wheat Sproat Chromatin and Involved in the Control of Cell Proliferation: Characterization by Infrared Spectroscopy and Mass Spectronmetry, *Peptides,* Nov; v.26(11): 2074-2085. http://www.sciencedirect.com/science/article/pii/S0196978105001786.

Hagiwara, Yoshihide. *Green Barley Essence.* Lincolnwood, IL: Keats, a division of NTC/Contemporary Publishing Group, Inc., 1985.

Jensen, Bernard. *Chlorophyll Magic From Living Plant Life.* Escondido, CA: Bernard Jensen, D.C., 1973.

Kiefer, Dale, "Superoxide Dismutase, Boosting the Body's Primary Antioxidant Defense." Life Extension Magazine, June, 2006. http://www.lef.org/magazine/mag2006/jun2006_report_sod_01.htm.

Lai, CN. (1979). Chlorophyll: The Active Factor in Wheat Sprout Extract Inhibiting the Metabolic Activation of Carcinogens In Vitro. *Nutrition and Cancer,* 1(3):19-21.

Lai, CN, B. Dabney, C. Shaw (1978). Inhibition of In Vitro Metabolic Activation of Carcinogens by Wheat Sprout Extracts. *Nutrition and Cancer,* 1(1): 27-30.

Mae, Eydie. *How I Conquered Cancer Naturally.* Garden City Park, NY: Avery Publishing Group, Inc., 1992.

Meyerowitz, Steve. *Wheatgrass, Nature's Finest Medicine.* Great Barrington: Sproutman Publications, 2006.

Peryt, Bogumila, Joanna Miloszewska, Barbara Tudek, Maria Zielenska, Teresa Szymczyk. (1988). Antimutagenic Effects of Several Subfractions of Extract From Wheat Sprout Toward Benzo[a]Pyrene-Induced Mutagenicity in Strain TA98 of Salmonella Typhimurium, *Mutation Research/Genetic Toxicology*, Oct; v.206(2): 221-225. http://www.sciencedirect.com/science/article/pii/0165121888901644.

Peryt, Bogumila, Teresa Szymcyzk, Pierre Lesca. (1992). Mechanism of Antimutagenicity of Wheat Sprout Extracts, *Mutation Research,* Oct; v.269(2): 201-215. http://www.sciencedirect.com/science/article/pii/ 002751079290201C.

Ren, Huifen, Hideaki Endo, Tetsuhito Hayashi.(2001). Antioxidant and Antimutagenic Activities and Polyphenol Content of Pesticide-Free and Organically Cultivated Green Vegetables Using Water-Soluble Chitosan as a Soil Modifier and Leaf Surface Spray, *Journal of the Science of Food and Agriculture,* v.81(15): 1426-1432. http://onlinelibrary.wiley.com/doi/10.1002/jsfa.955/abstract?userIsAuthenticated=false&deniedAccessCustomisedMessage=.

Savage, Candace. *Prairie: A Natural History.* Vancouver, British Columbia: 2 Greystone Books a Division of Douglas and McIntyre Publishers Inc., 2011.

Seibold, Ronald. *Cereal Grass, Nature's Greatest Health Gift.* New Canaan, CT: Keats Publishing, Inc., 1991.

Shah, Shinil (2007), Dietary Factors in the Modulation of Inflammatory Bowel Disease Activity, *MedGenMed,* v.9(1): 60. http://www.ncbi.nlm.nih.gov/pmc/articles/PMC1925010/.

Singh, N., P. Verma, B. R. Pandey. (2012), Therapeutic Potential of Organic Triticum aestivum Linn. (Wheat Grass) in Prevention and Treatment of Chronic Diseases: An Overview, *International Journal of Pharmaceutical Sciences and Drug Research*, 4(1): 10-14. http://www.ijpsdr.com/pdf/vol4-issue1/2.pdf.

Swope, Mary Ruth, and David A. Darbro. *Green Leaves of Barley, Nature's Miracle Rejuvenator*, Lone Star, TX: Swope Enterprises, 1998.

Szekely, Edmond Bordeaux. *The Essene Gospel of Peace, Book Four, the Teachings of the Elect.* USA: International Biogenic Society, 1981.

Wigmore, Ann. *The Wheatgrass Book.* Wayne, NJ: Avery Pub. Group, 1985.

Wigmore, Ann. *Why Suffer, How I Overcame Illness & Pain Naturally.* Wayne, NJ: Avery Pub. Group, 1985.

Yi, Bitna, Hiroshi Kasai, Ho-Sun Lee, Yunkyeong Kang, Jong Y. Park, Mihi Yang. (2011). Inhibition by Wheat Sprout (Triticum aestivum) Juice of Bisphenol A-Induced Oxidative Stress in Young Women, *Mutation Research/Genetic Toxicology and*

Environmental Mutagenesis, Sept; v.724(1-2): 64-68.
http://www.sciencedirect.com/science/article/pii/S1383571811002063.

Salty Minerals From the Oceans

Batmanghelidj, F. *Obesity Cancer Depression, Their Common Cause & Natural Cure.* Falls Church, VA: Global Health Solutions, Inc., 2004.

Brummit, Chris, "Tsunami Actually Aided Crops in Indonesia." USAToday.com, September 26, 2005.
http://www.usatoday.com/news/world/2005-09-25-tsunami-crops_x.htm.

Hendel, Barbara, Peter Ferreira . *Water & Salt, The Essence of Life.* Switzerland: Gymona Holding AG, 2002.

Landais, Emmanuelle. "Researchers Explore Ways to Use Sea Water for Farming." Gulfnews.com, Nov.23, 2010.
http://gulfnews.com/news/gulf/uae/environment/researchers-explore-ways-to-use-sea-water-for-farming-1.711262.

Langre, Jacques de. *Sea Salt's Hidden Powers.* Asheville, NC: Happiness Press, 1994.

Moyer, Melinda W. "It's Time to End the War on Salt," *Scientific American*, July 8, 2011.
http://www.scientificamerican.com/article.cfm?id=its-time-to-end-the-war-on-salt.

Mullen, Leslie. "Salt of the Early Earth," *Astrobiology Magazine*, June 11, 2001.
http://www.astrobio.net/exclusive/223/salt-of-the-early-earth.

Murray, Maynard. *Sea Energy Agriculture, Perfect Natural Nutrition?* Winston-Salem, NC: Valentine Books, 1976.

Newcastle University. "Ancient Oceans Offer New Insight Into Origins of Animal Life," ScienceDaily. September 9, 2009.
http://www.sciencedaily.com/releases/2009/09/090909133020.htm.

Ocean Health - http://www.oceanplasma.org/.

Ocean Solution Mineralizer – http://www.oceansolution.com/.

"Oldest Fossils Reveal Life 3.4 Billion Years Ago," *CBCNews, Technology and Science.* August 22, 2011. http://www.cbc.ca/news/technology/story/2011/08/22/science-oldest-fossils-bacteria-sulphur.html.

SeaAgri, Inc. SEA-90 100% Natural Sea Mineral Solids—Soil, Crop, and Livestock Nutrients from the Sea. http://www.seaagri.com/.

The Seawater Foundation. Sea water farming. http://www.seawaterfoundation.org.

University of California – Davis. "When the Earth Dried Out," *ScienceDaily*, February 8, 2002. http://www.sciencedaily.com/releases/2002/02/020208075438.htm.

Villemez, Jason, "Cotton Replaces Rice in Japan's Salt-Soaked Fields." PBS Newshour, September 16, 2011. http://www.pbs.org/newshour/updates/world/july-dec11/cotton_09-16.html.

Walters, Charles. *Fertility From The Ocean Deep, Nature's Perfect Nutrient Blend For The Farm*. Austin, TX: 2005.

Young, Gordon. The Essence of Life—Salt. *National Geographic*, September 1977, Page 381-401.

Soil

Brinton, W.F., Storms, P., Blewett, T.C. Occurrence and Levels of Fecal Indicators and Pathogenic Bacteria in Market-Ready Recycled Organic Matter Composts, *Journal of Food Protection*, Volume 72, Number 2, February 2009, p.p. 332-339(8). http://www.ingentaconnect.com/content/iafp/jfp/2009/00000072/00000002/art00 013.

Carson, Rachel. *Silent Spring*. New York, New York: Houghton Mifflin Company, 1962.

Darwin, Charles. *The Formation of Vegetable Mould Through the Action of Worms*. 1881.

"Fecal Coliform as an Indicator Organism," New Hampshire Dept. of Environmental Services, Environmental Fact Sheet, 2003.

Jensen, Bernard. *Empty Harvest*. Garden City Park, NY: Avery Pub. Group Inc., 1990.

Logan, William. *Dirt: The Ecstatic Skin of the Earth*. New York: W. W. Norton & Company, 1995.

Lowenfels, Jeff, Wayne Lewis. *Teaming with Microbes*. Portland, OR, Timber Press, Inc., 2006.

Nardi, James. *Life in the Soil: A Guide for Naturalists and Gardeners*. Chicago, IL, The University of Chicago Press, 2007.

Nutrition

Douglas, William Campbell. *The Raw Truth About Milk*. Panama, Rhino Publishing, 2007.

Fallon, Sally. *Nourishing Traditions, The Cookbook that Challenges Politically Correct Nutrition and the Diet Dictocrats*. Washington DC: New Trends Publishing, 2001.

Fife, Bruce. *Coconut Cures*. Colorado Springs, CO: Piccadilly Books, Ltd., 2005.

Price-Pottenger Nutrition Foundation - Dedicated to teaching the value of traditional diets for achieving optimal health in the modern world. http://ppnf.org/.

Price, Weston Andrew. *Nutrition and Physical Degeneration*. La Mesa, CA: The Price-Pottenger Nutrition Foundation, Inc., 2008.

Weston A. Price Foundation – The goal of this foundation is to restore nutrient-dense traditional foods to human diet through education, research, and activism. http://www.westonaprice.org/.

Good Oils

Budwig, Johanna. *Flax Oil as a True Aid Against Arthritis, Heart Infarction, Cancer and Other Diseases*. Vancouver, Canada: Apple Publishing Company Limited, 1994. (Seven time Nobel Prize nominee, Germany's foremost expert on fats and oils.)

Enig, Mary. *Know Your Fats: The Complete Primer for Understanding the Nutrition of Fats, Oils and Cholesterol*. Silver Spring, MD: Bethesda Press, 2000.

Enig, Mary & Fallon, Sally. *Eat Fat Lose Fat*. New York, NY: Penguin Group, 2005.

Fife, Bruce. *The Coconut Oil Miracle*. New York, NY: Penguin Group, 2004.

Glorious Wheatgrass Awaits You

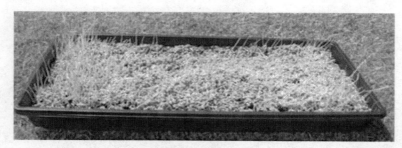

With the right wheatgrass growing supplies and this tutorial, say "good-bye" to poor batches of wheatgrass.

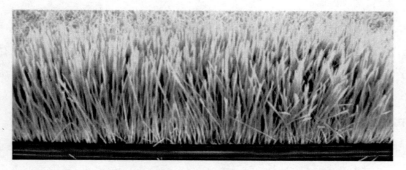

It's time to start growing thick, luscious, and nutrient abundant wheatgrass....

To a Healthier Tomorrow, One Sip at a Time....

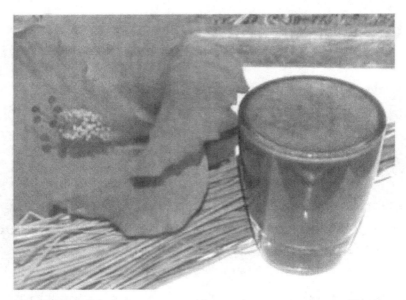

Awe, there is a great reward from your wheatgrass growing success. Nature's rolling grasslands grown in mineral and trace element rich soil feed the grazing animals superlatively well so they can be healthier.

Through consuming wheatgrass, a nutritional leader in the entire grass family, you can also directly access this fortifying food source. Just like fortunate grass-fed animals, I anticipate you too will be healthier from consuming your glorious wheatgrass juice—a supremely healthful grass-based gift from Mother Earth.

Replenish, Revive, and RELIVE, Cheers!

Visit the author at:

www.HealthBanquet.com

www.facebook.com/HealthBanquet

www.twitter.com/HealthBanquet

Sign up for Eryn's free Health Banquet Digest newsletter at www.HealthBanquet.com

Please leave a review at Amazon.

Closing Quote

K now, also, that the angel of Love is present in the blades of grass, for love is in the giving, and great is the love given to the Sons of Light by the tender blades of grass."

—Edmond Bordeaux Szekely
The Essene Gospel of Peace (Book Four)

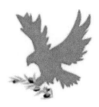

CPSIA information can be obtained at www.ICGtesting.com
Printed in the USA
LVOW11s1022110714

393925LV00002B/22/P